Praise for Hayley Hobson

"Learning to manage thoughts and emotions is life-altering. Applying what we learn from our insights and taking massive action produces results. Hayley Hobson is living her life in the way most of us dream about. Listen to her direction; she knows the way. I highly recommend you follow her lead."

—**Brooke Castillo**, Author and Master Certified Instructor

http://www.TheLifeCoachSchool.com

"Hayley Hobson is a MASTER at making things happen and getting things done. You owe it to yourself to dig in and learn from her. If you're seeking success and looking for some guidance...she's been there and done it, and she can lead you there."

—**Todd Falcone**, Author, Coach, and Speaker

http://www.ToddFalcone.com

"Hayley Hobson applies laser focus when helping people identify challenges, move past their fears, and take action in the direction of their dreams. She's a 'no excuses' coach who will stand beside you as you become the best that you can be."

—**Eric Worre**, Founder of Network Marketing Pro

http://www.Networking

T0125691

"Hayley keeps it real and makes it look like fun. This book will motivate you to clean up your act and make room for great things."

—**Desiree Rumbaugh**, Yoga Teacher and Author

"There are few network marketing leaders that are as results driven as Hayley. Her leadership style is direct and her stories hit you at your core. She is the builder's builder... not just a doer but a teacher! She travels the globe helping network marketers grow their teams. I have learned from her and you will too!"

—**Jordan Adler**, Author of the Amazon Bestseller, *Beach Money*

"I lived my life one extreme to the other until I read Hayley's book and realized I could have best of both worlds. I was either going 100 miles an hour supposedly 'getting it done' OR I was organized to the nines but accomplishing nothing. I now do both! This book truly changed my life!"

—**Tom Chenault**, Host of World's Largest MLM Radio Show

"Are you ready to elevate your life? Do you want to work/play at a level you didn't even think possible? If so, you need to partner with Hayley Hobson! Hayley is a perfect example of how to MAKE THINGS HAPPEN. She is driven, determined, knowledgeable, and accepts no excuses. Boom."

—Traci Porterfield, Former VP, Tony Robbins

"It's easy to believe that successful people are somehow cheating a system to which the rest are captive. Seize this opportunity to hang out with Hayley as she invites you to turn your headspace (the real source of captivity) into heart space. Let her simple yet profound 31 chapters serve like an a la carte menu where your heart selects the next meal to nurture your capacity to GET IT DONE!"

—Laura Jacobs, Speaker, Author, Holistic Health, Life, & Business Coach, doTERRA Presidential Double Diamond

Published by Mango Publishing Group, a division of Mango Media Inc.

Cover, Layout & Design: Morgane Leoni

For permission requests, please contact the publisher at:

Mango Publishing Group
2850 Douglas Road, 3rd Floor
Coral Gables, FL 33134 U.S.A.
info@mango.bz

For special orders, quantity sales, course adoptions and corporate sales, please email the publisher at sales@mango.bz. For trade and wholesale sales, please contact Ingram Publisher Services at: customer.service@ingramcontent.com or +1.800.509.4887.

Get It Done: Thirty-One Ways to Release Your Inner Boss

Library of Congress Cataloging
ISBN: (p) 978-1-63353-790-3, (e) 978-1-63353-791-0
Library of Congress Control Number: 2018946827
BISAC—SEL021000—SELF-HELP / Motivational & Inspirational

Printed in the United States of America.

GET IT DONE

Also By Hayley Hobson

A Beginner's Guide to Essential Oils

GET IT DONE

31 Ways to Release Your Inner Boss

Hayley Hobson

Mango Publishing

CORAL GABLES, FL

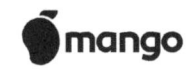

To all the women who have decided to make a shift in their lives and taken action to make it happen.

To those who have decided to courageously step up and step into the shoes of the new woman they wish to become.

And to those who have said, YES, there is a better way!

Contents

Introduction

Whoa. Before you go any further, if you were thinking this was a typical self-help book and that I am going to spoon-feed you success principles, well, that's not going to happen. No hand-holding either.

Well, maybe a little.

It's time to take charge. And if you need a little push, I'm sharing these *thirty-one ways to release your inner boss.* Your inner boss is powerful and supportive and there when you need her.

Now is the time to connect with her if your life is complicated, chaotic, or disorganized.

I'm crawling right into the mud with you to discuss what it will take to dig you out. You can choose to close this book and walk away, or you can step forward and make things happen.

No more excuses!

I know life can be tough. We all have challenges. Are you willing to allow those stumbling blocks to trip you up, or will you line them up and create the path to freedom? You can go either way. It's up to you.

I want you to have what you want, and releasing your inner boss will help you get there. I wrote this book to support you, but I can't do it for you. When it comes to your life, you're the boss.

Think fast and breathe slowly. You'll get where you want to go.

It's your choice from here. You can stop reading right now and gift this book to a friend, you can read from cover to cover and forget about it, or you can use it as a guide to *get it done*.

I hope making changes is your decision. Once you decide, you cut off access to any other options.

Where you go from here is your choice. There are millions of directions to choose from.

I'm going to ask one thing of you before we begin, though... Be honest with yourself. If you see yourself in one of these thirty-one chapters, be willing to look at what you see without judging yourself. Cut yourself some slack—nobody's perfect! Awareness is the first step to creating lasting change. Want to get it done? Open your mind.

Are you with me? Let's climb on this horse and ride!

XO,

Hayley

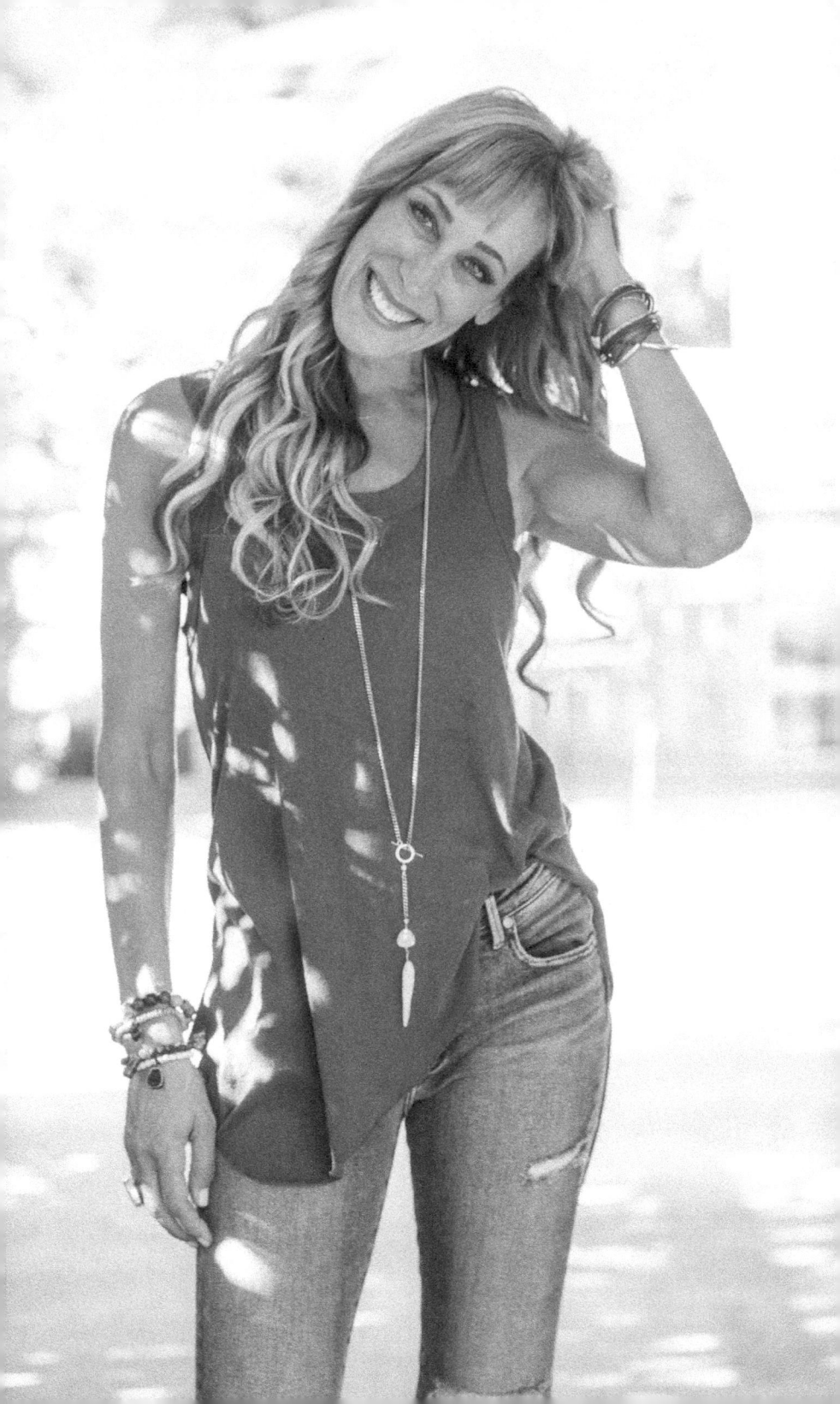

It's Your Job

Before we go too far, I'm going to come clean about a few things.

I lead a very busy life managing my home, a successful business, and a coaching practice—oftentimes from my phone. Yep, my phone. It's my office away from home. I thought I had created a system to help me balance my life, but as it turned out, I did just the opposite.

For a while, it worked. I got a lot of work done, and my business grew because of it. But instead of using my free time to rest or be with family, I worked.

The more I got done, the more I added to my plate.

My lifestyle was healthy and I had a lot of energy, but I was slowly wearing myself out. As I wrote this book, I remembered a realization I had during this stressful time that pretty much shocked me.

I had become addicted to the technology that was supposed to free me to live the kind of life a seven-figure annual income affords. Instead, I found myself a slave to my email, social media messages, and phone calls—and

I'm not talking just nine to five. I'm saying around the clock and even on weekends.

Low-level anxiety had become my way of life. Anytime my phone beeped, alerting me to a message, it flared like a flame in a sparkler factory. I couldn't let messages wait without an answer. This was partly because of my desire to please people and partly because answering my messages relieved my anxiety.

I used to blame others for messaging me at all hours of the day and night until I realized it was my accessibility that had given them permission in the first place. I've since learned to set boundaries.

I stepped to the front of the line by respecting those boundaries myself. I set specific times for checking and responding to messages, and I let everyone in my life know what those boundaries were.

Guess what? I don't blame anybody anymore. I am the boss of me, and managing my life is my job. I am responsible for taking control. Just like you are.

Is there an area of your life where you need to set boundaries? Are there any self-respecting adjustments in order? Think about what you would change and how you would change it.

Sometimes change (even positive change) brings on anxious feelings. Those anxious feelings are generated by anxious thoughts. The good news is you can change your thoughts any time you want.

What would your life look like if you took control? Well, guess what? It may not feel like it now, but you are already in control.

The *thirty-one ways* that follow offer a framework for making positive changes in your life. Some will be familiar, and other ideas will be new. You don't have to tackle them all at once. One step at a time will take you where you want to go.

Get it done

_____

_____

_____

_____

_____

_____

_____

_____

_____

_____

_____

_____

_____

_____

_____

_____

_____

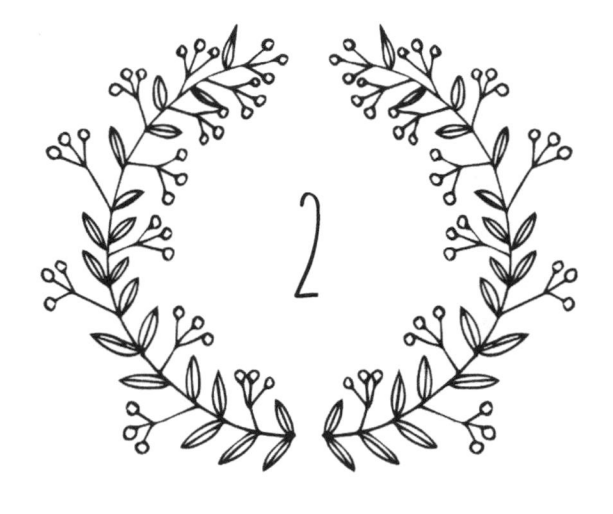

Get Organized

Stop Leaving Life to Chance

After you sort out your doubts and decide to make the necessary changes, your next step is to work toward organizing your life. Getting organized means different things to different people. Sometimes it means finding a place for things. Alternately, the process can involve digging out of wall-to-wall hoarding, pitching everything in sight, and then realizing later you needed and should have kept some of it.

Like everything else, organization begins in the headspace. If your thoughts are organized, your life will be organized. Organization is about creating harmony and balance in your life. It means aligning your actions with your purpose.

What if your whole life is disorganized? Well then, you go around in circles. You can also think of it like riding bumper cars. You have to be hyper-vigilant—watching and trying to avoid collisions while making sure everything doesn't spin out of control when you turn your head.

Already feeling out of control? You have two choices:

1. Be organized and prepared.
2. Respond to life as it unfolds.

I've done it both ways. Guess which is easier?

How can YOU begin organizing your life?

After organizing your headspace, the next step is organizing your environment. Even if it's a corner of a room, define a space that is yours alone and build from there.

Here are a few hints.

ORGANIZING YOUR WORKSPACE

For me, being organized begins with having an orderly workspace. Everything has its place, and I know where stuff is when I need it. This is really important because as a "momtrepreneur," an organized workspace is the foundation for *getting it done*. All of it!

My workspace and home are organized in a way that makes life comfortable and easy for me. I'm not compulsive, but I attribute much of my success to staying organized.

I know that everything trickles down from the top, so when my own life is balanced, my family's lives are more balanced, too.

Okay, tell me if you can relate. Does life sometimes feel like a juggling act? Me too. If I were not organized, everything would probably fall apart. I would be living in CHAOS—unable to manage my time or my tasks.

FILE INSTEAD OF PILE

We all know people with big piles on their desk. They say, "Don't worry. I know where everything is. I can find it when I need it."

Yeah? Maybe....

If you're a piler, you might *think* your organized mess is efficient, and you might know what papers are in which piles, but try to imagine what it would be like if you developed a filing system. What would it be like to know exactly where to look for what you need? You'd feel less anxious when you have to find something in a hurry, wouldn't you? You only have to create a system you can follow, and it only takes a few extra minutes to put things away as soon as you're finished with them.

Disorganization, on the other hand, has several drawbacks. It can be the source of invisible tension, affecting your mood even though you might not be fully aware that it is where the problem started.

Disorganization affects you emotionally. It can be super stressful! And again, that stress is there whether you're consciously aware of it or not.

If you're a piler, your life will be changed overnight by developing a filing system. Give it a try and see. From there, it just takes discipline as you create a new habit. Eventually it will be automatic.

List Makers Unite!

Okay, so there are average list makers and then there are serious LIST MAKERS. Average list makers write all of their tasks on one to-do list and work from it. Serious LIST MAKERS break tasks down and create categorized sub-lists. Sometimes they're pages long.

Go with what works for you.

Be patient. I'm going to spend a little time on this subject because list making is a valuable aspect of being organized.

Besides helping you stay on task, list making has other benefits. Let's discuss some of them.

First of all, if you commit to a list, you won't have to worry about forgetting things at the market or mailing letters so long as you list them with your daily tasks. Write it, do it, and cross it off. Bam!

By the way, it feels really good to cross off completed tasks. In fact, some list makers add completed tasks to their lists just so they can cross them off. There's a reason for this. It's both psychological and physiological.

The reason it feels so good to cross off completed tasks is because to some degree you're after the natural high that follows.

You've heard of endorphins, right? They're brain chemicals that are released internally and react with the opiate receptors in the brain. They act in pretty much the same way as morphine or codeine. Well, endorphins are released every time you cross completed tasks off your list. Jolt! Endorphins are powerful, so get ready. We will discuss them again later on in the book.

GET STARTED LISTING

As noted, you might prefer to write everything on a single master list. Or, depending on your responsibilities, it might work better for you to divide business and personal tasks between two separate lists:

1. A personal to-do list
2. A business tasks list

You might think this is going overboard, but some people find it easier to make separate lists for everything: shopping lists, domestic tasks lists, business tasks lists, and Honey-Do lists. (That last one is the one you give your spouse or kids to be sure repairs and other chores get done around the house.) If you choose the multi-list method, be sure to keep your lists together so you can stay organized.

If you're not familiar with list making, do what comes easiest for now. You can always refine your system later.

The purpose of listing is to stay organized, not to feed your OCD, so be sure to create a system you feel comfortable with. Guidelines are simple. Just write in a stream of consciousness.

Write down all the tasks you need to complete in the order they occur to you. Remember to list projects, errands, and decisions you need to make.

Once you've written down every task you can think of, minor to massive, categorize tasks according to the system you created. This is easiest if done on your computer. Create a Word document, or if you are comfortable with Excel, create a spreadsheet. A timeline-style listing might work for you.

Long-Term Goals

List your dreams and aspirations—for the year and way down the road.

Monthly Goals

Monthly goals don't necessarily come with a sense of urgency but may have to be completed during the month or repeated every month; paying bills, for instance.

Weekly Goals

What do you need to accomplish in a week's time? Grocery shopping, appointments, weekly meetings....

Daily Goals

These are activities and tasks you need to complete every day. Exercise, take supplements, uh, call Mom.

You might want to have a category for your social gigs. Things like soccer games, recitals, and girls' night out may involve reprioritizing in other areas.

Organizing Email

A ton of correspondence is done by email for most people these days. Depending on how active you are on email, you could receive anywhere from five to several hundred emails a day.

And how many do you *send*? I'm not talking about mass email blasts. I mean the one-offs. Go back and count them sometime.

It might be a good idea to set up two separate email accounts: one for business and one personal.

In the business account, create master files for major categories.

For example, I have files for:

- Leads
- Follow ups
- Events
- Travel (I even break this down monthly and by trip)

- Company
- Team
- Products
- Marketing
- Subscriptions
- Confirmations

Create your own digital system and e-files for whatever applies to your life and business.

Scan your email every day; when an email comes in, file it in one of the master files. If it helps, you can also have sub-files in any category.

Minimize stress by organizing your life. My husband Wes is always asking me where his wallet is, where his keys are, where his glasses are....

I know where everything of MINE is.

My purse is always in the same place, and all of my cabinets are or-gan-ized! Even the drawers in my bathroom are organized. And I don't hang on to stuff I don't need. I cleanse every few months. That means getting rid of anything I have not used in a while!

Ready? You try. What one simple aspect of your life can YOU organize immediately?

If you work at organizing in small pieces, you'll make it happen. Come up with your own arrangement. It'll provide a solid platform on which to build your success.

Begin today with ONE THING. Get it done!

All good? Good. Let's keep going.

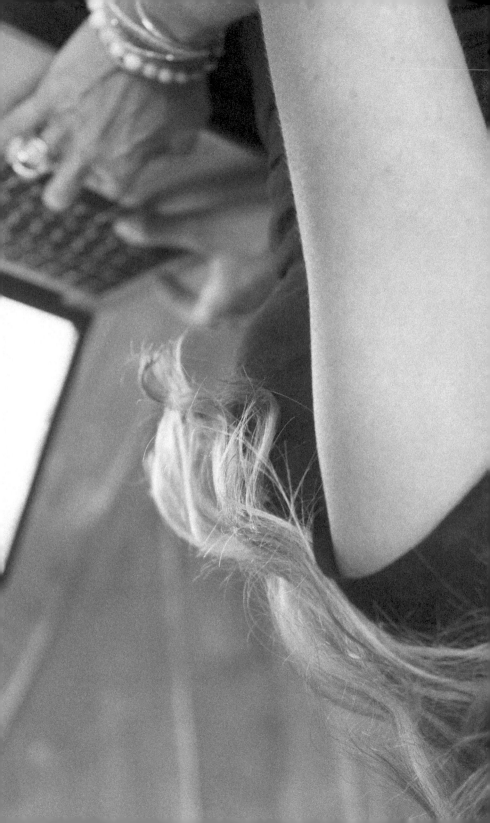

Get it done

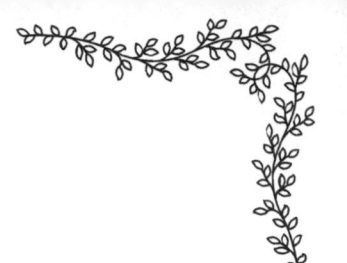

_____

_____

_____

_____

_____

_____

_____

_____

_____

_____

_____

_____

_____

_____

_____

_____

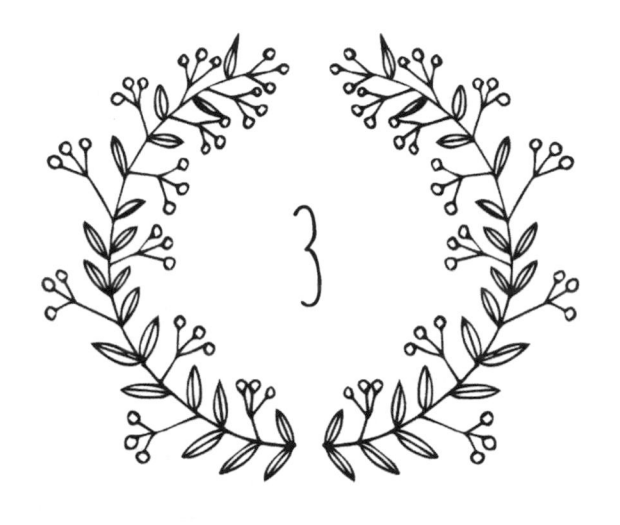

3

Let Go and Make Space

Emotionally, Mentally, and Physically

Making space means more than cleaning out your closet or selling a few broken toys or worn-out sweatshirts at a yard sale. Now, it's still important to rid your living space of clutter, so don't get attached to Grandma's end table. But for our purposes, making space also refers to inner space.

That's where you start. Out with the old, in with the new.

Making space will give you room for more of what you want. While you're de-junking your environment, grab a shovel and dig out of the mind clutter you've been hanging onto. It's been weighing you down, and the time has come to get over it. Clear your mind and focus on the tasks at hand—like taking the first steps to fulfilling that dream of yours.

Now, I'm not totally without sympathy. It's super easy to become snowed under by life. It can feel like falling into a deep hole you'll never get out of.

Seriously, think about everything you do in a single day.

If you tracked every task you completed from the time you roll out of bed until you turn off the lights at night, you'd probably be shocked by how much you actually do. You'd also probably wonder how the heck you manage to get all of it done.

Well, when you *sometimes* get it all done.

Sometimes you don't.

Those don'ts can add up and be right there staring you in the face the next day. What happens? Your list gets longer and the stress mounts. All that unfinished business leads to one thing...CHAOS!

Craving Alone Time?

Want to know a secret? I'm going to tell you something a lot of moms feel guilty admitting. (Not me.)

I LOVE my alone time. And I don't always get enough—do you?

Some of us crave solitude, but in today's world, it's hard to get away from people. I am not just talking about Facetime. Between our cell phones, texting, email, and other forms of communication, there's nowhere to hide.

Remember what happened to me. Technology seems to be taking up more space every day, and in the process, pushing us out of the way. All those devices and apps converge to make things tighter.

Who's da boss? You. MAKE SPACE!

Make Space for Wellness

Wellness involves more than a yearly physical. It's also more than exercising and eating healthy. Mental and emotional stability are just as important, and clearing your mind is an important aspect of mental balance.

I come from a holistic viewpoint that takes into account mental and social factors, rather than just the surface definitions of wellness. When you MAKE SPACE in your life and think positively, your emotions are more likely to respond in kind.

How do you make space? Here are a few suggestions.

ABOUT THAT CLOSET....

Not ready to tackle this topic yet? Okay, forget the closet for now.

Let's begin with something you're less attached to: the junk drawer.

Almost everybody has a junk drawer, right? What's in yours? There might be tools, tape, matches, batteries, and things you might need at some point. There might also be paper clips, hair ties, and old sticks of gum. Junk drawers are the place you throw things that have no home.

Be honest with yourself. Some of that stuff can go straight into the trash, right? "I might need it some day" is an excuse for holding on. All it does is complicate your life.

Pick a day to tackle the junk drawer. Empty it completely and throw away anything you've mentally labeled, "Things I might need some day." If you haven't used an item in six months, toss it!

Okay, Time's Up! About That Closet

Time to breathe. This one can be tough. Our closets are sacred! We can be attached to the contents. Hey, I know people who've kept clothes in their wardrobes for a decade or more. They keep shopping and stuffing in new clothes, and pretty soon they can't find anything.

I have a little empathy. I'm the first one to shop for new clothes and accessories. But I also pass things along if I'm not using them.

Just as you did with the junk drawer, pick a day to deal with your closet. Before you begin, set ground rules and promise to honor them. Work with a friend who will hold you to the mark. Prioritize and then decide what to keep and what to give away.

Dig in! You never know what you're going to find. I know someone who was brave enough to exhume the dead weight from the back of her closet, and you know what ended up in the giveaway box? Her $2,000 wedding gown. She'd been married twenty years, and there was no reason to keep it other than sentimentality.

She said she remembered how much fun she'd had playing dress-up as a kid, and since she had no daughters, she gave the dress to Goodwill. The thought of some young woman feeling like a princess had more value to my friend than hanging onto a memory.

So, take a deep breath...and purge!

MAKE SPACE IN YOUR INBOX

Are you an email hoarder? If you have Gmail, you've found the email hoarder's best friend. Gmail has a super huge storage capacity for years of emails. And if you use it up, for $1.95 a month you can buy more. Yep, an email hoarder's dream come true.

It might be tempting to hold on to emails in case you want to refer to them in the future, but think of your inbox as a virtual junk drawer. Muster your courage...MAKE SPACE!

Read it, file it, or trash it.

LIMIT SOCIAL MEDIA ENGAGEMENT

It's easy to get lost in social networks—just like shopping. You might run into the market for apples and come out thirty minutes later with two gallons of juice and a bag of veggies. If you're hungry, maybe three!

My point is this: whether your go-to faves are Facebook, Twitter, Instagram, or Pinterest, you can get totally lost and forget what you visited for. It's easy to lose track of time perusing social media.

I know you know what I'm talking about. Have you ever logged onto Facebook to check your notifications and then come out of a trance realizing forty minutes have passed? You can waste hours meandering around groups and websites and cluttering your mind.

If this happens to you often, set limits. Set an alarm when you go online. It'll make you aware of the passage of time. And don't hit the snooze button!

When it comes to surfing the internet, watching YouTube, or burying your face in your Facebook newsfeed, self-discipline is your only salvation.

RELEASE NEGATIVE EMOTIONS

Holding on to negativity takes up emotional space. Why carry your pain around? Make space by releasing negative emotions such as bitterness, anger, and resentment.

Resentment is super toxic. It's the process of repetitively replaying feelings of anger or rewinding mind-movies of events that brought the negativity about in the first place. By doing so, you force yourself to relive experiences emotionally, mentally, and even physically.

Regardless of whether you are hurt or angry, allowing the actions of another to occupy your heart and mind only hurts you. The only way out is to release. It may seem as though you're doing it for the other person, but you're actually doing it for yourself.

FORGIVENESS

The word *forgive* doesn't mean "let the other guy off the hook" or "sweep it under the carpet." It could mean, "bury the hatchet," but not in the other person's back, of course!

"Forgive" actually translates as "to free." The Greek translation means "to let go." Letting go frees emotional space and it comes with HUGE health benefits as well.

Begin by forgiving yourself.

Whether we're aware of it or not, we all hold onto resentment toward ourselves for our own mistakes, certain behaviors, and slip-ups we make.

Subconsciously, resentments set off a chain reaction. First, they cause us to judge ourselves harshly, and then that judgment calls for punishment. These judgments are often the source of feelings of being undeserving and self-sabotage. Self-sabotage can affect everything you do for the rest of your life—unless you deal with it.

Let go!

Regardless of what has happened to you, whether by your own hand or that of someone else, release it. Don't let anger occupy space in your heart or head.

The value of making space in your life extends far beyond the space itself. When you release, let go, and move on, you open up more of what the *good* life offers. Make space for life, love, and happiness!

Get it done

_____

_____

_____

_____

_____

_____

_____

_____

_____

_____

_____

_____

_____

_____

_____

_____

4

Prioritize

What Comes First?

How are you doing so far? Getting the hang of things? Everything I discussed in earlier chapters comes together here:

- Organizing your life requires a system
- Making space is necessary for organizing
- AND prioritizing is an aspect of making space

If *getting it done* is your goal, knowing your priorities and following through is the best way to achieve what you're after. I'm taking for granted that you have the idea and you're ready for the heavy lifting.

Whatever your priorities, be sure they're in alignment with your goals. If they aren't and you're out of whack, you can always move things around and sync them up.

Now, don't go criticizing yourself because of your priorities! A priority is something that's important to *you*, and everyone's priorities are different. It's a personal thing. We prioritize for our families, businesses, and other relationships, and for every aspect of our lives.

Well, at least we prioritize in our heads. Have you taken the time to prioritize on paper? Really! It makes a difference in *getting it done.*

Your family might be the most important focus in your life. I know mine is. Maybe your career heads the list. Knowing what you want most will help you align what you do with your priorities.

If you're single, you will probably have different priorities than someone in a relationship, with or without kids. Some singles focus on building their careers and others on shaving their schedules down to a four-hour workweek. Whatever your center of attention, there's no right or wrong—it's up to you.

You might be a relationship person. Which relationships are your priorities? Is spending time with your longtime friends most important, or are you into meeting new people? How about dating? Prioritizing will allow for balance and harmony between all the facets of your life.

So Much to Do!

At times it can seem like the world is crashing down on top of you. If you're a mom, you have a major responsibility. In

45

traditional families, there's the house and a family to care for, unless you can afford to hire help. If you have littles, there's school, as well as homework, doctor's appointments, playdates—you know the drill. And if you're a single parent, most of it falls on you, the chief cook and bottle washer.

If you're a "momtrepreneur" and run a business, it can be especially hard to get everything done. I know this firsthand.

Between my travel schedule, webinars, and private coaching, I work super hard to keep my life balanced.

I have to keep things going at home while managing my professional life. Sometimes it seems like meetings, paperwork, communication, training, and education have to be squeezed in between other responsibilities. I won't let non-priorities take precedence or allow my family to suffer because of them.

Even super important things can slip between the cracks if you're not paying attention. Do what you can do and then somehow find a way to pick up the slack.

Learning to prioritize effectively will help you be more efficient by helping you get to the most important things first. It'll save time, and in the process, energy. The bonus? LESS STRESS!

First, dig all of your priorities out of your head and commit them to paper. Even if you have a great memory, we're working on making space, so holding things in your head is counterproductive.

Here are a few tips to help keep you aware of your priorities so you can place them at the top of your to-do-now list.

PULL OUT YOUR TASK LIST

As I wrote in the first chapter, making monthly, weekly, and daily task lists will help you organize everything you need to accomplish in each of those time frames.

I know you're busy. I'm busy too. But you'll be glad you took the time to do this exercise. It might seem unnecessary, especially if you're used to keeping everything in your head, but trust me, there's value.

Order by Priority

Identify the most important or urgent tasks on your list by using a number or letter system:

1. Most Important
2. Important
3. Least Important

Put the corresponding number next to each item on the list: (1) most important, (2) important, and (3) least important. Then rewrite the list in order of priority. Again, depending on your top priorities, family activities might be at the top of the list. Projects and errands might be next. It's your list. If many things are equally important, choose randomly. What matters is that you get things done.

Keep your list accessible and visible. Use it as a reminder of what needs your attention.

Get it done

_____

_____

_____

_____

_____

_____

_____

_____

_____

_____

_____

_____

_____

_____

_____

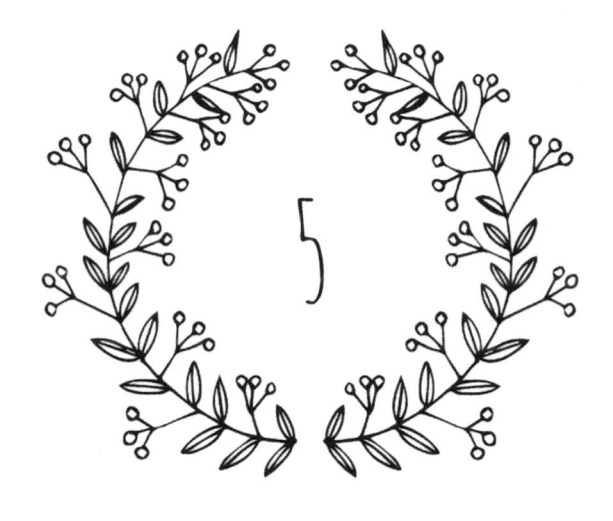

Goal Setting

Map It Out, Write It Down, and Dive In!

Goal setting. Hmph. Okay, I saw you roll your eyes.

LOL—I actually agree with what you might be thinking.

Goal setting is probably the most oversaturated topic of discussion ever. Does that mean it's not important? Of course not! In fact, it's probably the most important skill you can master, and that's why I've included it as one of the *thirty-one ways to release your inner boss*.

Before we go any further, I have to say that if you're not already setting goals—or not willing to set them, go right ahead and close this book. And don't put it on your bookshelf either—get it out of the house altogether. Put it with that box of stuff going to Goodwill (remember, the one from your closet) or give it to a friend, and go back to your life as it is.

I'm being very serious when I say that goal setting is a skill you must master, because if you're going to rely on blind luck to create your future, you're committing to a life of confusion and chaos. You might as well pack it in right now. Without goals, your life will be no more than a crapshoot. YOU are too important and too valuable to settle for that.

And when you're finished reading this chapter, can I ask you to do one more thing? Set at least ONE goal. Jump on my Facebook page and tell me what it is, or join my group, Consciously Creating Your Whole You with Hayley Hobson.[1]

Deal?

Cool! I can't wait to hear from you so I can support you.

Goals get a bad rap, you know. It's not so much goal setting that's difficult; it's meeting the goals we set that can be challenging. No one said you have to be perfect. Commit! Move past those sticky obstacles and go after what you want. Accomplishment will lead you right onto the path of success.

Wait a sec. You can go *too* far.

The biggest obstacle to success is setting monster goals. These are goals that are so complicated you avoid them altogether. Resist the urge.

---

1 Find more information at:
   https://www.facebook.com/groups/consciouslycreatingyourwholeyou/

Set yourself up for success instead of standing in your own way—because if you don't step aside, some of your heart-held goals will likely never become reality. Start with achievable goals first and then move on to more complex goals.

Short-Term Goals

Begin by setting short-term goals. These goals require less effort and manifest quickly. Short-term goals usually encompass a variety of categories and occur over a relatively short period of time—hours, days, or up to a month.

What would you like to get done by the end of the day? By the weekend? Do you have errands to run before you pick up the kids from school? All of these are short-term goals. Accomplishing them will allow you to string together a series of successes that will inspire you to keep going.

Try this: use a system of setting short-term goals to support you in accomplishing long-term goals when you break them down into manageable, doable steps.

Long-Term Goals

Long-term goals are goals you have to work at, or goals that take time to bring to fruition.

> *Where would you like to see yourself a year down the road?*
>
> *What are your ambitions for the future?*

These are the goals you work toward. They require a little elbow grease and often involve several smaller activities to make them happen.

Long-term goals require planning. If your goal was to get more education or training, one of the top priorities would be to clarify what you want to learn. After you figure that out, choose how you will get that training. Gathering the resources to pay for that training would probably be at the top of the list.

Other long-term goals might be to start a business, quit your job, take a cruise around the world, get married, buy a house....

Being willing to take action is a positive trait, but taking action without a strategy in place can be a waste of time. For this reason, knowing SPECIFICALLY what you want is super important. If you're not sure what you want, get sure before you set your goals.

Taking action before being clear about what goal you're moving toward is like taking a shot in the dark.

BRAINSTORMING IDEAS

Brainstorming can be used for both your short-term and long-term lists. Usually two or more people get together and bubble up ideas and thoughts.

Do you have a couple really witty friends? You know, those quick thinkers who are good with a comeback? Invite them over and then help each other brainstorm ideas.

You can also brainstorm by yourself. It's called "stream of consciousness." There are a couple ways to tackle this task. Grab a pen or open a text document on your computer. You can also use voice recognition software and let it transcribe your words.

GETTING WHAT YOU WANT

There are all kinds of goals. Be patient. Give yourself time to make things happen. It's important to set financial goals, personal goals, and if you're an entrepreneur, business goals. Again, know what you want and go after it.

What if you change your mind later? Fine! Change your goal.

Of course, you could just think about and dream about having what you want, but you'll probably only end up thinking and dreaming, not having. Or you could just close your eyes and point. You might hit your goal, and you might not. Open your eyes and make a plan and you're more likely to have what you want.

Is your goal attainable? Do you believe you can do it, have it, be it? If not, be open to changing your beliefs, because if you don't believe in yourself, you won't get there. There's just so far you can go on other people's belief in you.

Here's something to think about. Do you really want what you're going after? Does your goal excite you? If not, find a new goal. Your emotions have so much to do with dreams coming true. You really need to be motivated and willing to take action. If not, it will never happen.

Give your mind a target and then take aim. Be clear and specific.

When you choose a direction, here are a few questions to ask yourself:

When do you want it?

A year from now? Tomorrow? When your kids are grown and out of the house?

What will it look like?

Describe it. Come up with as much detail as you possibly can for your goal.

What do you need to get there?

Are there specific materials you need? Certain people?

Why do you want this goal to come to fruition?

What purpose will it serve?

Be sure to identify the markers that will help you know you're on the right track—and also those that will signal that you're not. How else will you know you've achieved your goal?

Your Timeline

All of the above questions—even with answers—have little value without making that plan we were talking about. Part of a plan is creating a timeline for the steps you'll take to make things happen. Your timeline has a starting point and ends with a deadline. The deadline can be fluid. You can change it if need be, but set one.

Trust yourself, friend! Set the bar higher than you think you'll be able to go. I promise you'll surprise yourself with what you're capable of. We often sell ourselves short. Dream big and then shoot for the friggin' moon!

Get it done

_____

_____

_____

_____

_____

_____

_____

_____

_____

_____

_____

_____

_____

_____

_____

_____

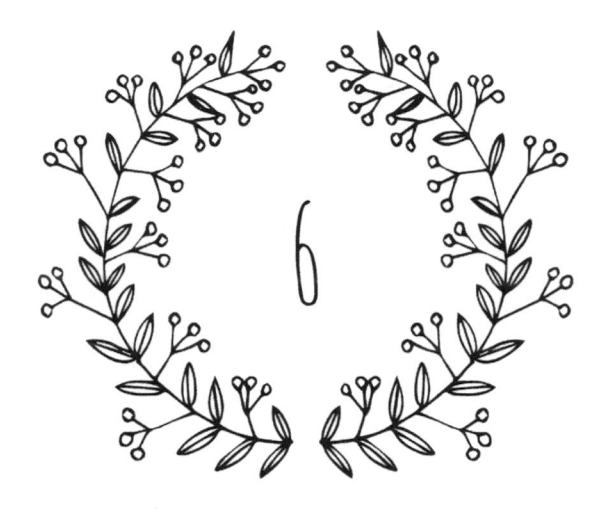

6

Dream Big

In Living Color!

Kids dream big. They see themselves as princesses, astronauts and other powerful figures. It's not until someone tells them they CAN'T that some kids believe they WON'T.

And then some don't ever believe in those limitations.

Be that kid inside, no matter how old you are or how BIG your dream is. You can dream anything you want, and keep in mind that dreams do come true. Dreamers have impacted history by committing to their visions no matter what anyone else believed was possible.

In your heart of hearts, you want to be happy. I know you do; we all do. At the core of happiness is true satisfaction with life. That's why even simple dreams have value.

It's thrilling when dreams come true. It can feel magical. Dreams can revolve around career, parenthood, or competency with a specific skill set. But whether or not dreams come true, they do not define us. They do, however, give dimension to our existence.

Dreams help us focus on our core values. Some people dream of finding a person to share their lives with; a spouse, a life partner, or even a best friend. Relationships are central to happiness, beginning with our most important relationship: the one we have with ourselves.

Financial dreams usually have something to do with prosperity, having the resources for comfort, pleasure, and self-care. When they come true, they also provide the ability to purchase material possessions we desire.

What are YOUR dreams? What do you want....

> *To Have?*
> *To Be?*
> *To Do?*

Does it feel like you're on your way to having what you want, or do your dreams seem out of reach? Don't let anyone tell you your dreams won't come true. You really can have what makes you happy. Dream BIG, because the bigger you dream, the more likely you are to get what you want.

You might be thinking, *Well, that doesn't make sense. Wouldn't it work better to keep my dreaming down to earth? I will be more likely to get what I want if I don't set my sights too high, right?*

Wrong! DREAM BIG, and then set smaller, achievable goals to make your BIG dream come true. When it does, dream bigger!

Examine Your Thoughts

What are you saying to yourself? Your thoughts create your reality. If you're telling yourself you will never have what you want, chances are you won't. Examine your thoughts! (More on this in Chapter 8.)

If you believe you're undeserving for whatever reason, you'll subconsciously push away every opportunity that could move you closer to your dream coming true. Your thoughts reflect everything you believe about yourself. If you "think" you're incapable, you tell yourself that. And then you believe YOU!

You listen to what your thoughts tell you is or is not possible. Examine your thoughts and then change the ones that hold you back.

For instance, if you think, "I don't have the money to..." you will make sure you don't. If you change that thought to, "I have the resources to..." you will always attract what you need.

Visualize

In 1978, Shakti Gawain published a tiny manual titled *Creative Visualization*. It's a skinny little book, but it made a huge impact and ushered in a new way of thinking about manifesting what you want and making dreams come true. It's still on the market forty years later.

The book teaches how to use mental imagery and affirmation to bring about what you want by first visualizing, or "seeing it" in your mind. By creating a vision and then a mind movie, you can bring your dream into reality. I've done it many times.

About 60 percent of us actually see pictures in our minds. Some of us see them in color. If you're among the 40 percent who do not, does that mean you can't use the creative visualization process? It does not.

You can use your imagination.

For example, imagine what it's like to see yourself living your dream. You might not see the actual pictures, but you can feel what it's like. Attach emotion to it. How does it feel to have what you want? I imagine it feels pretty good!

Ignite Your Emotions

As you visualize or imagine your BIG BEAUTIFUL DREAM being achieved, you will feel awesome. Get excited! Open your heart and feel the joy! You're telling your unconscious mind exactly what you want, and it will respond in ways that will astound you.

Really enjoy the feelings of success and gratification that come with this simple exercise. And remember to express gratitude. Thank yourself, thank life, thank God—or whomever/whatever you wish. Gratitude always brings more of what you're grateful for.

Energize Your Vision

A popular activity among those who believe in energizing visions is creating a vision board or dream board. This is a pictorial depiction of dreams, goals, and intensions. There are many possible forms; for instance, you can use a large piece of foam core or cardboard to display your visions, or create a three-ring binder or a spiral-bound book. It doesn't matter how you do it as long as you create a visual image of your BIG DREAMS.

Affirm Your Big Dream

I've heard people say affirmations don't work. I disagree. Whether positive or negative, they work, and they help to bring about whatever they're associated with.

Positive affirmations will work in your favor when you:

- Use them consistently.
- Keep saying them until you believe them.
- Use them properly.
- Associate them with feelings and use appropriate language.

Always dream big, friend. You're worthy of your heart's desire, whatever it is. And you're never ever stuck. You can also change your mind anytime you want.

Believe in your ability to make things happen, and don't wait for your dream to drop into your lap. Take action!

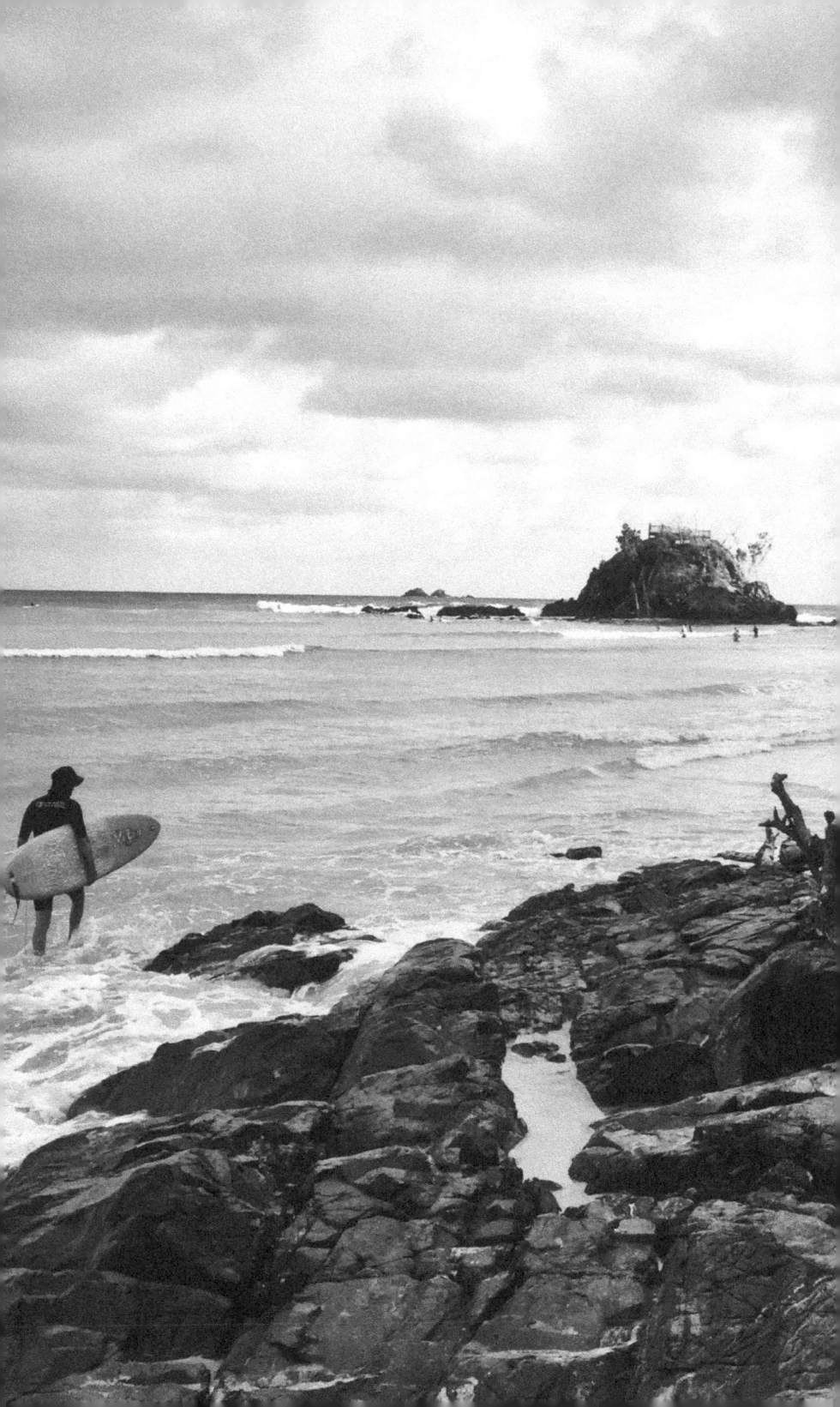

Get it done

_____

_____

_____

_____

_____

_____

_____

_____

_____

_____

_____

_____

_____

_____

_____

_____

_____

_____

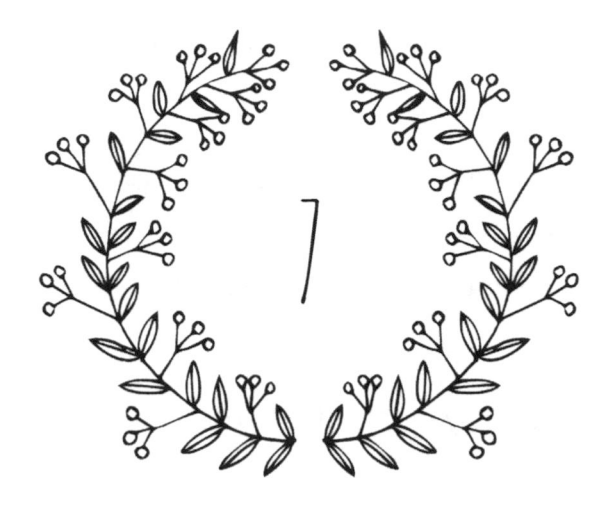

Author Your Life

Rip Up All Other Scripts

There are people who live their lives making someone else's dream for them come true while their own dreams wither and die.

Sometimes children grow up to please parents, or build careers others want for them. Even as adults, they can be unaware that they've allowed other people to author their lives.

Do you know anyone like that? I do!

ME!

I lived the first half of my life trying to please others. I busted my behind in law school to become an attorney, something I never really wanted for my life. It was one of the most miserable times of my life, even though I did it well for five years.

One day, I had the courage to walk away from my successful practice and six-figure annual income. I had no clue what the future held. From that time forward, I have been authoring my own life, and I have been happier than ever before.

Authoring your life means living the life YOU want to live. You take what you've been given to work with and make it better. It means doing the best you can to BE the best you can.

What it would be like to look back someday and see that your life had gone in a direction that was of your dreams? Can you imagine if you'd never said or done the things you dreamed you would? It would be heartbreaking, right? You can't go back in time.

It's time to write your own script. Author your own life, and never allow anyone else's expectations to influence the direction you take. Don't let your parents, society, or your significant other—or even your kids—tell you what you should or shouldn't do with the time you have on this earth. This is YOUR life!

Do you want to be happy? I KNOW you do. What will it take? The most important question is—are you willing to do the friggin' work? I hope you don't have to think twice to answer.

The first thing you need to know is what your dream life looks like so you can go after it.

71

You're not married to your choices, and you can change your mind whenever you want. In fact, count on life changing direction more than once. The more you grow and evolve, the better acquainted you'll be with who you are, and the surer you'll be about what floats your boat in life.

Explore each of these areas:

Mental

Education, knowledge, training, career focus, personal and professional expression (books, blogs, teaching, etc.)

Emotional

Love, friendship, partnership, resolution, healing

Physical

Health, wellness, exercise, body image, etc.

Spiritual

Religious practice, meditation

As with everything, you may encounter challenges. Some you'll have control over and others you won't. It can make you crayballs! Here are four keys to finding balance and moving past perceived barriers so you can begin authoring your life.

Remember Those Goals?

We talked a little about goals in Chapter 5. Your goals will probably change as you evolve. Go ahead and add, delete, or adjust goals anytime. Authoring your life means describing how you'd like each aspect of your life to look and feel. What do you see when you look into the future? Set your unconscious mind free and write whatever comes—without censoring.

DEFINE YOUR STEPS

Take a blank sheet of paper or open your laptop and write what you want at the top of the page. Let your ideas flow and write out steps you can take toward having the life you want. List baby steps and granddaddy leaps—short-term and long-term goals.

TAKE ACTION

Hang on a sec. Setting goals, visualizing, and writing affirmations are valuable tools, but like I keep saying, they are pretty much worthless unless you take action. The more action you take, the faster you'll get what you want.

Every time you take a step, no matter how small, you'll feel a sense of accomplishment that will energize you.

BE OPEN-MINDED

Yeah, so you're playing with the big dogs now. Most people are unwilling to go this far. They'd rather stick with what's comfortable and familiar than open their minds and step into the unknown.

Take it from me; you never know what the Universe is going to throw at you. The most valuable way to support yourself in authoring your own life is to keep an open mind.

You're going to discover things about yourself you didn't know were there.

You'll unearth the best of who you are.

You'll also dig up stuff you are ready to dump. Good. Dump it. Everything serves its purpose, and if you're done...let go.

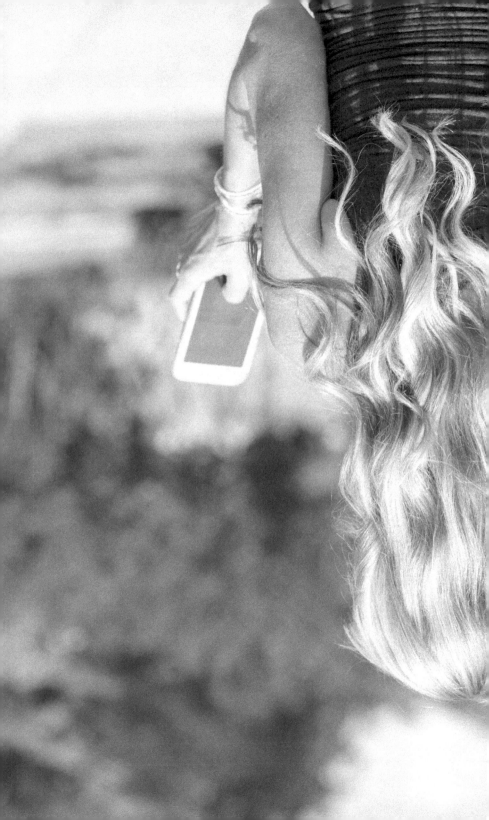

Get it done

_____

_____

_____

_____

_____

_____

_____

_____

_____

_____

_____

_____

_____

_____

_____

_____

_____

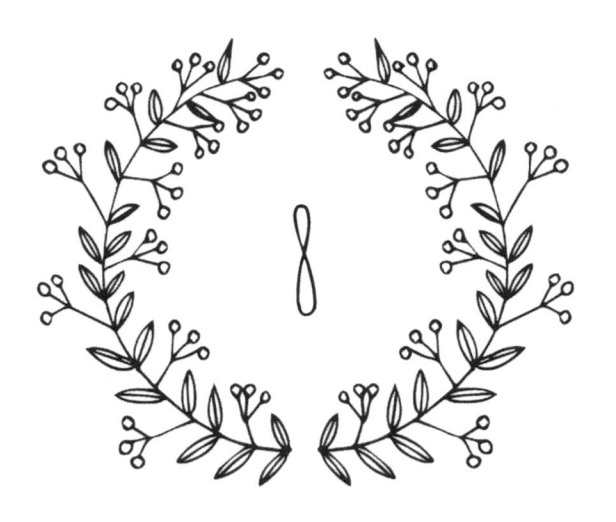

Pay Attention to Your Thoughts

So, what have you been cramming between your ears lately? You can bet it's a lot more than you realize. Did you know you have 70,000 thoughts a day? That's forty-eight thoughts per minute! You don't remember everything, but that's what passes through your mind.

This can (and often does) take you off track.

Your thoughts create your reality, so if you're feeling frenzied, examine what's been occupying your headspace. It's not only *what* you think; it's also *how* you think it that matters. If you're out of sorts, you can restore balance by CHOOSING different thoughts.

Out of everything you hear, you listen most intently to your own SELF-TALK. This is the stuff you tell yourself about yourself and the world.

It doesn't matter what others say. What YOU think, you believe before anything else. If you internalize what others say, it becomes self-talk, and that's massively risky.

Your belief system dictates what you think is possible. In order to reach your full success potential, you must learn to believe in yourself.

Regardless of appearances, know unequivocally that you are capable, competent, and deserving of success! Don't let anyone tell you otherwise!

But there's far more to life than believing in yourself and positive affirmations. Once in a while, allow yourself to choose a thought that simply makes you feel better.

If my husband doesn't call me when I'm traveling, I'll choose to believe he's still sleeping, doing something with the kids, or just busy. I don't believe that *he doesn't love me because he doesn't call*. Someone else may choose to believe, "What a jerk, he never calls."

In my business, a lot happens on the last day of the month. That used to piss me off. I used to think, "Why can't people get things done sooner? Don't they care?" Now, I just choose to think that everything will happen the last day of the month. And with that thought, I no longer have any expectations, and that calms me down.

There's no point in creating scenarios in your head that might not even exist. Don't assume and let your mind run wild. All that does is cause unnecessary pain. You'll drive yourself cray-cray.

Thoughts and Goals

Trusting in your ability to reach your goals will allow you to have thoughts that support your efforts. Think about it...you've already accomplished tons of things, right? You have amazing qualities that enable you to go after—and have—what you want. But first you need to believe you have those qualities, and when you do, don't keep it a secret. TELL YOURSELF.

Even if you don't believe (yet), the more you remind yourself that you are positive, hot, and successful, the more you'll begin to see yourself this way. Others will too. You'll exude confidence. Believe you are beautiful and then watch everyone else begin to tell you that you are.

While you're at it, how about making a little space for a few more positive thoughts? It's easy. Begin by releasing negative thoughts. (Remember the chapter on making space? Yep, that one.)

Many people are experts at talking themselves down. They think less of themselves than others do and then act in ways that prove their points. Thinking that bad things always happen to you will attract bad things!

Think life is not fair? Guess what? Life will not be fair.

Think there's no way you could earn a six-or-seven-figure income, and guess what again? You won't.

That's how powerful your thoughts are.

As long as you watch your thoughts and allow positive thoughts that support your success, you'll get what you want—sometimes more. You don't even need to know HOW to accomplish your goal. Just believe it is possible and keep telling yourself you will get it.

Can I tell you what the only thing standing between your success and you?

It's YOU.

It's the same with releasing your inner boss. Change your thoughts and change your experiences. Instantly.

Get it done

_____

_____

_____

_____

_____

_____

_____

_____

_____

_____

_____

_____

_____

_____

_____

_____

_____

Honor Your Feelings

The feeling of inner imbalance can be highly charged and emotional, and your emotions can go in several different directions at once. It can be exhausting. Anxiety and frustration head the pack.

In the same way you need to pay attention to your thoughts, it's important to notice your feelings. This comes with being self-aware.

Now, did you notice I didn't say, "act on your feelings?" That's a whole other subject. In fact, much of the time you want to do anything but act on your feelings.

Your feelings are reactions to things going on around you. They are a form of communication between the mind and body.

When an event happens, or when you see or hear something, you react with emotion. Certain reactions are automatic. Other times you can control your feelings. But even with feelings you can't control, you can learn to manage how you express them.

Some people don't recognize what they're feeling because when they were young, their feelings were not validated.

When they cried, their parents may have told them there was nothing to be sad about, or when they were angry, they may not have been allowed to cry. People who grow up this way often don't recognize what they're feeling as adults.

Do you take the time to notice what you're feeling? Are you in tune with your emotions?

There are four basic emotions: mad, sad, glad, and scared. If you have trouble recognizing how you feel in a situation, ask yourself one by one, "What am I feeling: Mad? Sad? Glad? Scared?" Because these are basic feelings, you will more easily recognize feeling at least one of them. You can train yourself to recognize feelings.

Positive Attitude

Is a positive attitude an emotion? Well, not really. But a positive attitude dictates some of your thoughts and feelings. An attitude is a position—an outlook or perspective.

Have you ever heard that positive people see the glass half full and negative people see the same glass half empty? Same glass, same amount of water—different points of view.

The person who sees the glass half full might be happier. Happier people get more done. It's easier to calm yourself and bring yourself back into balance if you're positive.

The person who sees the glass half empty might be scared, sad, or angry because of his or her interpretation. Negative peeps may say they are merely being realistic. It doesn't matter. Being positive is more productive than being negative, no matter what's going on.

YOU can choose to be positive. You can decide to approach life with the intention of getting things done, and you know what? You will!

Get it done

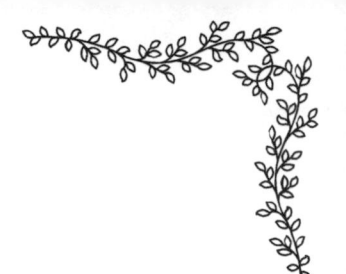

_____

_____

_____

_____

_____

_____

_____

_____

_____

_____

_____

_____

_____

_____

_____

_____

_____

_____

10

Observe Your Actions

Without Self-Judgment

You've probably heard the old adage, "Actions speak louder than words." It's true. Actions are the outward expressions of our thoughts. Learning to think fast is an asset.

Your thoughts lead to feelings, and feelings lead to actions. Observe your feelings and then your actions. Feelings either motivate or de-motivate you.

How are you responding to what is going on around you?

One of the most valuable things you can do is:

THINK GOOD THOUGHTS

If you're having negative thoughts, change them.

FEEL GOOD FEELINGS

If you're angry or sad, honor the feeling and move on.

TAKE DETERMINED ACTION

Take a deep breath and step forward in the direction of your dreams!

Is your life chaotic? As I mentioned earlier, chaos can bring on confusion. If you're confused, you'll be less productive. Balance will elude you. Observe your thoughts and actions and be determined to change them when they stand between you and what you want.

Center yourself. Restore balance mentally and emotionally and your actions will reflect your inner world.

Don't give up!

What would it look like for you to be relentless in your commitment to move through obstacles and challenges? Close your eyes and imagine those roadblocks dissolving. Walk straight through them toward peace and balance.

You have the ability to do this. Use it! All it takes is practice, and then in time, it'll come naturally.

Get it done

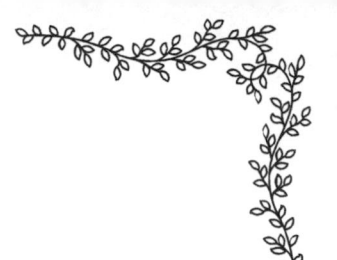

11

Schedule Everything

Don't Trust Your Memory

I know, you're sure you can keep track of everything. Even if you have a photographic memory, I'll go out on a limb and suggest you can't. Schedule everything—write it down.

If you don't keep track, something will fall through the cracks, guaranteed, and if it's super important, you may not be able to recover from the backlash.

I see this happening to people around me every day. They agree to meet or plan a phone call, but they don't write it down. Then they forget. Sometimes they're granted forgiveness, but at other times, they ruin relationships or lose out on opportunities altogether.

This happens often in my business. People schedule appointments with me and then come late or don't show up at all. I have to wonder how much importance they place on our meeting. Are they really just forgetting or are they blowing it off altogether?

The truth is, with my busy lifestyle, I could be one of those people if I tried to commit everything to memory. Even if

I jotted an appointment down on a piece of paper to add to my calendar later, I might forget to add it. What then?

If I'm the one picking up my daughter at the bus stop, I schedule it, because honestly, I can get so lost and absorbed in work that if I didn't schedule it, I'd forget. And then that face...ugh, when she walks home all by herself. Not good.... Bad mama.

I actually get a little crazy neurotic about it. Like, if I have a flight at 1:20 p.m., I schedule the flight. Then I backtrack and schedule the bus I'm taking to the airport from downtown Boulder. Next, I schedule the time when I'll have to pull my car out of my own garage and leave for the bus stop. That way I get reminders for everything. "Hayley, leave the house or you'll miss your friggin' flight." I love that!

I need to live a stable life. That's why I schedule every meeting, every phone call, every errand—everything. My integrity is too important to risk letting things collapse.

I hate to think of what would happen to all the balls I'm juggling if I dropped one because I was irresponsible.

Are you success-conscious? If you're success-conscious, the one thing that will sabotage your future success will be flaking on appointments.

If you prefer analog systems to digital, buy a planner and USE IT. I can't tell you the number of people I know who spend a ton of money on expensive organizers and then go through the year having barely used them.

Commit to using your planner for thirty-one straight days.

Observe what happens.

Does digital work better for you? There are a number of scheduling apps out there. Choose a system that works for you, or you won't use it. If you have a Google calendar, use that. There's a lot you can do to record appointments and activities daily, weekly monthly, and beyond. You can even set up alerts to remind yourself to remind yourself.

Schedule everything. It doesn't matter how you do it.

Down the road, there may be things that become routine, like taking the kids to school, but in the beginning, write down even the most mundane tasks. (And if you need to keep things like this on your calendar to avoid scheduling calls during that time period, do it.)

If scheduling is challenging at first, don't stress. You'll get better as you go along. Doing something for thirty-one days straight helps to create a habit. Once scheduling is ingrained in your body-mind system, it becomes automatic.

Decide How Much Time You'll Spend on Specific Activities

It's easy to miscalculate the amount of time necessary to complete specific tasks. Let's say you have three 30-minute phone meetings on Wednesday morning, starting at 8 AM. I would not recommend scheduling your calls back-to-back to the minute.

Here's why...

Things don't always go as planned. If you schedule your first call from 8–8:30 AM and your second call from 8:30–9 AM, one of two things could happen:

1. Your first call might go over, even by a minute, and you'll be late to your second call.

or

2. You'll end up rushing your first call to avoid being late for your next appointment.

Thirty minutes is not a long time. Whoever you're meeting with deserves your full attention—don't give them the shaft.

Give yourself five to ten minutes between calls just in case.

MEETING IN PERSON

Some people actually still meet face-to-face. Can you believe it? I'm being sarcastic, but depending on how old you are, you may have grown up in a world where most everything is done online, over the phone, or via Skype. Before technology expanded our options, most people met in person.

If you have a face-to-face meeting or an event to attend, make sure to account for travel time. Leave extra time in case of traffic, car trouble—or even plain old "being behind schedule" stuff. If it's smooth sailing, you might arrive early. Wait in the parking lot if your appointment is scheduled at a specific time. Use the extra time to check email or handle some biz. Or do something you might forget to do because you're so busy—RELAX.

YOUR DAILY CALENDAR

What do you do every day without fail?

> *Check email?*
>
> *Pick someone up?*
>
> *Work out?*

Calendar these things and stick to your schedule. Plan your exercise time, meditation time, specific household chores, or any other activity you do on a regular basis. Your weekend calendar might look different than your mid-week calendar. Create a daily outlook for both.

Don't leave your schedule open for appointments ALL DAY LONG. Why? Because you are NOT available all day long. You have other commitments, either to yourself or others.

You have to go for a run, or head to a yoga class, or record a podcast or webinar, or put together some images for social media, or write a blog, or meet someone to discuss your business or product, or pick up your kid, or eat.

So SCHEDULE all of that and then choose the time blocks you want to be available to book calls to build your business. Not in business yet? Maybe it's time to schedule that call to explore the idea!

Schedule Mental Health Breaks

Be sure to schedule time for yourself! No matter how much you love what you do, taking time to chill will energize and revitalize you. You need time to fill your own cup. How you spend that time is up to you, just make sure you're resting your body and mind. Schedule it or you won't do it. If you schedule it into your day, you'll consider it a priority.

Breathing techniques and yoga can help you relax. (See the chapter on yoga and learn about benefits.) Schedule regular vacations, even mini vacations. You don't even have to leave town if you don't want to. Check into an upscale hotel and pamper yourself. Not only do you deserve it, your emotional, mental, and physical health depend on it.

Be sure to schedule the end of your workday—especially if you work from home. You might think it's totally doable to close the door to your office and let go until the next day, but it's not always easy. Your business doesn't always leave your mind just because the clock says it's quitting time. Schedule it. End your day at a reasonable hour, and honor your agreement to yourself.

Keep Promises

When you set an appointment, keep it. That includes phone meetings.

Now, stuff comes up for all of us. That's life. But unless it's an absolute emergency, keep your appointments. Even if you have to cut the meeting short, show up. Set a new appointment or make an amendment to show the person their time matters.

When you blow off appointments—whether you forget or just don't show—you say something about yourself. You send a message (or two) to the person you were supposed to meet with: you are disorganized, or worse, the meeting was not important to you.

If you make a habit of flaking or forgetting, it will undermine your success and impact your relationships. Here are a few tips to keep you on schedule.

SCHEDULE PERSONAL REST BREAKS

If you don't schedule them, they may not happen. Some people even have to schedule meals and snacks or they forget to eat.

PUT TIME ASIDE FOR THE UNEXPECTED

We all know stuff happens. Especially if you have young children or other family members to look after, things pop up. Unless you have a nanny or support, leave some flexibility in your schedule.

BREAK DOWN LONGER ACTIVITIES

Instead of blocking out a huge chunk of time in your calendar for longer activities, assess whether they can be broken down into smaller pieces of time.

Success-conscious people lead busy lives, but successful people manage their lives. They don't miss appointments—telephone or otherwise—and they don't blow things off.

Schedule everything and you will not fall short on keeping commitments—and you'll also relieve yourself of a huge amount of stress.

An important part of this conversation is to avoid overscheduling so you can manage your life. The next chapter will shed some light on this subject.

Get it done

_____

_____

_____

_____

_____

_____

_____

_____

_____

_____

_____

_____

_____

_____

_____

_____

_____

_____

_____

12

Ask for Help

You Don't Have to Do it All by Yourself

Are you a doer? Most entrepreneurs are. You have the kind of get-up-and-go that motivates you to get things done. If you didn't, you'd be okay with following all the sheep building someone else's dream.

Even if you're still a 9-to-5er, if you're an entrepreneur at heart, this won't be okay for long. Either way, here's something to remember: There is a thin line between being a doer and a do-it-all-yourselfer. Read that last word carefully because this trait is present in almost every novice entrepreneur until they learn otherwise. Many new entrepreneurs think they have to do it all, and do it alone.

We all get overwhelmed from time to time. With too much to do in too little time, we start thinking about everything that's going to fall apart if we don't bring everything back into balance.

Ask any entrepreneur and most will tell you they've been there at one time or another. Some who've learned to outsource aspects of their business still find themselves battling the *do it all* syndrome. It's not an easy thing to unlearn, but once you do, you'll wonder why it took you so long.

The Great Juggling Act

Most entrepreneurs live multifaceted lives. We are partners, parents, friends, business owners, and more. Every one of these roles requires time and effort to do well. It's easy to overcommit, overschedule, and overdo. Have you noticed this in your life?

You juggle all of it and keep doing everything until it becomes too much. This kind of lifestyle comes with a very expensive price tag. In the beginning it might work, but after a while, it can rob you of the most valuable thing you have: quality of life.

You do all this to avoid feeling guilty for needing help. Well, guess what?

Eventually you'll do everything half-assed and end up shrouded by guilt—guilt that you're not giving your loved ones what they need because of your business, and guilt that you're not giving your business all the attention it needs because of your family responsibilities.

How do you handle a multitude of responsibilities without going crazy? Here's how....

Set Boundaries

This one can be tough—especially if you're a "momtrepreneur." You might not even know what this would look like in your life, let alone how to do it. Not only do you have family activities, but your business also needs attention. It's easy to become overwhelmed.

Boundaries are the lines you draw in the sand—the lines you should never allow anyone to cross. Granted, the boundaries we have with our families are a little more flexible than those we have with others, but it's important to set boundaries and honor them.

Learn to say no. This can be a huge challenge—especially for women. We think we can do it all, and we often can, but overscheduling only leads to stress and exhaustion.

You're in charge. You teach people how to treat you.

Remember to set boundaries with yourself, too, and respect them. Every time you honor your boundaries, you get better at doing it the next time. It fosters self-respect. The better you get at it, the more you can trust yourself to take care of yourself.

I Need Help

Do these words bother you? Some people feel if they can't do it all by themselves, they're somehow second-rate. Do you ever feel that when you can't get everything done by yourself you're somehow incompetent or less than other people who seem to have it all together?

You're not.

Things aren't always as they appear on the outside. I guarantee that if you know a highly successful person who appears to be managing a busy life easily and effortlessly, something is giving somewhere. Either that or they've learned how to ask for help.

What does it mean to ask for help?

Well, once you handle overcommitment and have pared your life down to a manageable pace, asking for help can mean different things in different areas of your life.

HELP WITH THE FAMILY

Parenting can be a fulltime job. It doesn't matter how many kids you have. In fact, a bigger family is often easier to manage than if you have an only child. At least you have a ready built team to help do household chores and entertain each other. If you have one child, you're it. All of it, at once.

If you're a working parent, your workload intensifies. Try adding even 10 hours a week to an already full schedule. Your 8-hour day just went to 11 hours.

Asking for help with the kids doesn't mean you're a substandard mother. There is no shame in hiring a babysitter a few hours a week, even if it's only to go to Starbucks to chill for a bit. In fact, when you take care of yourself, you'll be an even better mom. There'll be a difference in the way you parent and the kind of partner you are, and your family will notice.

If you can afford a nanny, go for it. This option doesn't work for everyone, so if it's not your thing, stick with a part-time babysitter or swap playdates with other families.

Do-it-ALL-yourself mothers are sometimes critical of moms who get help. DON'T take on their shame. It's okay to ask for help! As long as you're spending quality time with your kids when you're together, and you can afford it, hiring support can work for you. That goes for a housekeeper too.

HELP WITH YOUR BUSINESS

This is one of my favorite things to talk about. Why? Because if you have a business in today's world, you've chosen the best time to be an entrepreneur. It's never been easier to own and run a business—never in history, and it's only getting easier.

Have you heard of outsourcing? Outsourcing is the practice of hiring contractors to help you manage the tasks involved in running your business. Do-it-ALL-yourselfers, don't get nervous. This is a super positive thing.

The reason many entrepreneurs feel they have to do everything themselves is because they think they are the only ones who can do it right.

Maybe that's true and maybe it's not.

But you'll never know unless you learn to trust. It takes a huge amount of trust to delegate responsibilities to other people. And you take on an equally huge responsibility when you are the one to whom the responsibility is being delegated.

The truth is, even if you know you are competent and can do something without help, if you're already doing too much, you won't be able to do everything well. Something will fall through the cracks.

If you outsource tasks to other competent people, you'll put your business on the fast track to success—financially and otherwise. Most importantly, by shedding all the operational and tedious tasks required to sustain your business, you will be free to enjoy the reasons you started it in the first place.

Let's talk about which tasks you can outsource and which are best kept within reach.

You might not realize it, but you're probably outsourcing already. Do you do your own accounting, or do you have a bookkeeper? How about your taxes? Do you file on your own, or do you hire a tax preparer? If so, you're outsourcing. Even if your brother-in-law does your taxes for you, you're still outsourcing. Whether or not he's competent or trustworthy or you just don't want to do it yourself, it still qualifies as outsourcing.

Any task you delegate to someone else is outsourcing.

Other tasks you can outsource are those you do not have the skills to do, don't want to do, or don't have to do yourself. These might include: writing, project management, appointment setting, communications, social media marketing, etc. Tasks that generate income directly are better kept close to home. Such tasks might include: networking, relationship management, and sales.

Make two lists and divide tasks you must do from tasks you can outsource. Remember, you can keep any task you enjoy. If you like working with numbers, go for it. Do your own bookkeeping. If not, by all means pass it along. Delegate the time you would have spent working IN your business and use it working ON your business.

Are You a Perfectionist?

If you're a perfectionist, the trait you value most might actually be the one that stabs you in the back. There have been many perfectionists who stop just short of their goals because what they're doing is just not good enough.

111

Good enough for WHOM?

Good enough for themselves.

If you put yourself through the wringer, it doesn't usually stop there. Perfectionists usually judge others just as harshly as they do themselves. Because of this, they think no one is able to do things as well as they can and they turn down help.

If this is you, I want to tell you circumstances will never be perfect.

There will be times you just have to settle for things as they are.

I know you don't want to live in chaos, and you don't have to. Accept help from others. Hiring someone to help with tasks can make a super big difference in your life and your stress level. Decide what to delegate and then let it go.

Some activities aren't worth your time. If the cost of your time outweighs the cost of hiring someone to help, cough up a few bucks and make a call.

A good boss knows how to delegate. Release her and find out.

Get it done

_____

_____

_____

_____

_____

_____

_____

_____

_____

_____

_____

_____

_____

_____

_____

_____

_____

_____

Be Vulnerable

This Means Being Authentic

Hey, life can be rough sometimes. It would be nice to think you can walk through it wearing fluffy bedroom slippers, but it's not always like that. I'm sure more often than not you feel like you have to trudge through with combat boots, right?

Just because you're a badass and the road is rocky, who says you have to be hardcore?

Being vulnerable means opening your heart when all you really want to do is close yourself off for protection. You don't have to navigate this world on your own. Allow yourself to be vulnerable. Graciously receive special care and support from others.

How does being vulnerable play out in real life?

We can't talk about vulnerability unless we first talk about walls. Do you put up walls to protect yourself? By walls, I'm talking about something you hide behind for protection; not letting people see the real you.

Walls can be tall and wide or they can be short. It doesn't matter. They serve the same purpose—they keep people out. They provide a false sense of protection that might defend you from attacks, but they also shield you from intimacy in your relationships.

Deep down, most people want to be real. They just don't want to get hurt, so they guard themselves and don't allow the door to their hearts to open too wide.

Being vulnerable is risky because it means putting yourself out there. It's wearing your heart on your sleeve. And yeah, you can get hurt. But healing the hurt that occasionally comes with vulnerability is better than cheating yourself out of the fullness of what can be when you let people see the real you.

Being real in your relationships will change your life. Allow yourself to risk with someone you feel safe with—a good friend or a new friend you're starting to feel close with. See what happens. I'm betting you'll bring out the "real" in your friend, too.

Relationships enrich our lives. When you choose healthy relationships, you'll feel safe being vulnerable, and others will feel safe with you. You'll not only see your best qualities reflected, but you'll learn what it's like to live with an open heart.

Get it done

_____

_____

_____

_____

_____

_____

_____

_____

_____

_____

_____

_____

_____

_____

_____

14

Cultivate and Nurture Your Relationships

Do you have a group of friends? Maybe you know a lot of people but have just a couple close friends? Whether you prefer one-on-one over a cup of coffee or being surrounded by an entourage anytime you leave the house, relationships are important. They enrich life and make it more beautiful.

There are all types of relationships—family, love, friendship, and other personal relationships. We'll go into those in a minute.

But first, let's get down to biz.

Business relationships are a special kind of relationship, and the success of your business depends on them. This chapter goes hand in glove with the previous chapter on networking.

Networking is only socializing unless you cultivate relationships, and those relationships have the most value when you nurture them.

Let's say you're a network marketer. (I am too.) You know that if you're going to build a team or generate income, you have to play a numbers game to promote and expand your business.

It's the same with any kind of sales business. If you sell anything—products or services—you're in sales, and that's also a numbers game. The more people you are connected to, the more likely you are to reach your numbers and build a successful business.

A word of warning: whatever you do, don't become a relationship-hoarder. It'll quickly be obvious if you're the kind of person who collects people just for the sake of putting them in your back pocket. Just plain don't do it. Be genuine, authentic, and willing to give and take. Your business will thrive.

PERSONAL RELATIONSHIPS

The cornerstone of relationships, business or personal, is mutual respect. It begins there and then grows into fondness and sometimes love. Loving relationships are like ice cream. There are a zillion flavors, but when you get down to it, they're all ice cream.

Cultivating friendships calls for maturity and responsibility. Along with respect and fondness, authenticity plays a major role. Be who you are and not who you think your friends want you to be.

Oh, and don't give to get. As each of your relationships deepen, the real you will eventually shine through. If you're hiding behind a mask, you can bet your friends will be shocked when it accidentally slips off—and trust me, it will.

Never change for others. Accept who you are, AS you are. Grant the same courtesy to your friends, and anyone worth your friendship will do the same.

Tell people how much they mean to you. It can be scary putting yourself out there because it opens you to rejection. But you know what? It can also help deepen intimacy with people you care about.

I didn't used to be comfortable doing this with people in my business, but since I moved past my fear, I've developed some unbelievable relationships. My lifestyle makes it challenging for us to spend a lot of time together, but I do let the people in my life know how special they are and how much I love and appreciate them.

I'll tell you something, those simple words go a long way, and your relationships will be super solid when you can step away from your ego and tell someone else how awesome they are. The love comes right through you, and expressing the way you feel feels great.

Get it done

_____

_____

_____

_____

_____

_____

_____

_____

_____

_____

_____

_____

_____

_____

_____

Develop Partnerships

With Likeminded People

The secret to productivity and efficiency can be partnership as long as you have the right partners. Successful businesspeople value their partnerships with likeminded people.

Ever watch *Shark Tank*? Many of the guest entrepreneurs say their partnerships with the multimillionaire or billionaire investors are more valuable than their financial infusion. I would agree.

MARRIAGE AND LIFE PARTNERSHIPS

Marriage is a partnership. Don't be such a badass that you don't put the work into a relationship you promised to fight for.

Just as with any committed love relationship, marriage and life partnership take tons of effort to make them work. They require megadoses of mutual respect and willingness to do whatever it takes. Whether or not a document makes it legal, if you commit, you commit. Mature relationships are not for the faint of heart, that's for sure.

Is life partnership worth all the energy it takes to sustain it? Well, that depends. Everyone is different. You might say there is nothing more gratifying than journeying through life with a significant other, or you might enjoy living single.

If you prefer a twosome, you can make a marriage work in such a way that is satisfying for both partners. Do this and you'll have accomplished a task that fewer than 50 percent of people who attempt it are able to do. Over half of marriages end in divorce.

A SUPER IMPORTANT POINT!

Okay, this is a touchy subject, but it's important to touch on. If your life partner or spouse is abusive in any way—emotionally, mentally, or physically—walk away. No one deserves abuse.

If you're really unhappy and have grown apart, try to make it work, and if you can't, you're cheating yourself and each other by staying in the relationship. If you have kids, you're also sending a message to them about relationships. Is it the message you want to send?

BUSINESS PARTNERSHIPS

It might surprise you to know that business partnerships are a lot like marriages and just as challenging to maintain. Equal partnerships, where both partners share the workload and rewards, must provide space for open communication. Each partner must learn superior listening skills and be willing to compromise. Like I said—reminiscent of marriage, right?

Healthy business relationships require a lot of maturity. Be really sure you are willing to go all the way or else don't do it. Just as in marriage, if something goes wrong and can't be repaired, a business divorce can be really painful and destructive to both partners.

OTHER PARTNERSHIPS

If a full business partnership is not your gig, there are other kinds of partnerships. Take the time to explore ideas. Partnerships can and do work when you're willing to do your part. They can be profitable when you partner with the right person or people. Take your time before jumping in.

Here are a few tips on creating mutually beneficial partnerships.

PARTNER WITH PEOPLE WHO SHARE THE SAME OR SIMILAR VALUES

What motivates you? Your values. Can you imagine what it would be like to partner with someone wanting to move in the opposite direction? Frustrating! It's like a game of tug-of-war, or push-me-pull-you. Two opposing viewpoints create two opposing sets of behavior and no one gets anywhere.

Set the Ground Rules in Advance

You create a business plan for a business, right? You set goals to bring that plan to fruition. It's just as important to set the ground rules for your partnerships. But guidelines have little value unless everybody knows the rules in advance.

Have Open Lines of Communication

Some say rules are made to be broken. Not. That's lazy and irresponsible. But it does happen. Whether intentionally or not, rules are broken, boundaries are violated, and mistakes are made. Life unfolds as it does.

Having open lines of communication is essential if you want to move toward a peaceful resolution, which comes with a willingness to listen. It means all parties feel safe in sharing thoughts and feelings without fear of retribution or punishment, so no ganging up on anybody, regardless of who agrees or disagrees with whom.

Here's a strategy you can try. Schedule regular meetings to discuss issues and concerns. Set ground rules so you can be productive in resolving issues. You can be informal. Pass an object around; whoever is holding it gets to speak while everyone else listens with no interrupting.

BENEFITS OF PARTNERSHIPS

A great thing about partnerships is that you get the benefit of diversity among partners. Everyone comes to the table with their own personal experience and areas of expertise. By yourself, you might have ten years of experience in a particular area or business. Add in the ten from your partner and it becomes twenty years. See the value?

Partnerships allow each person to learn from the other. The strengths of one partner can make the other partner(s) stronger. Partner with people who raise the bar and force you to stretch. Sure, it's gratifying to be the one who KNOWS, but it's more valuable to be the one who LEARNS and GROWS.

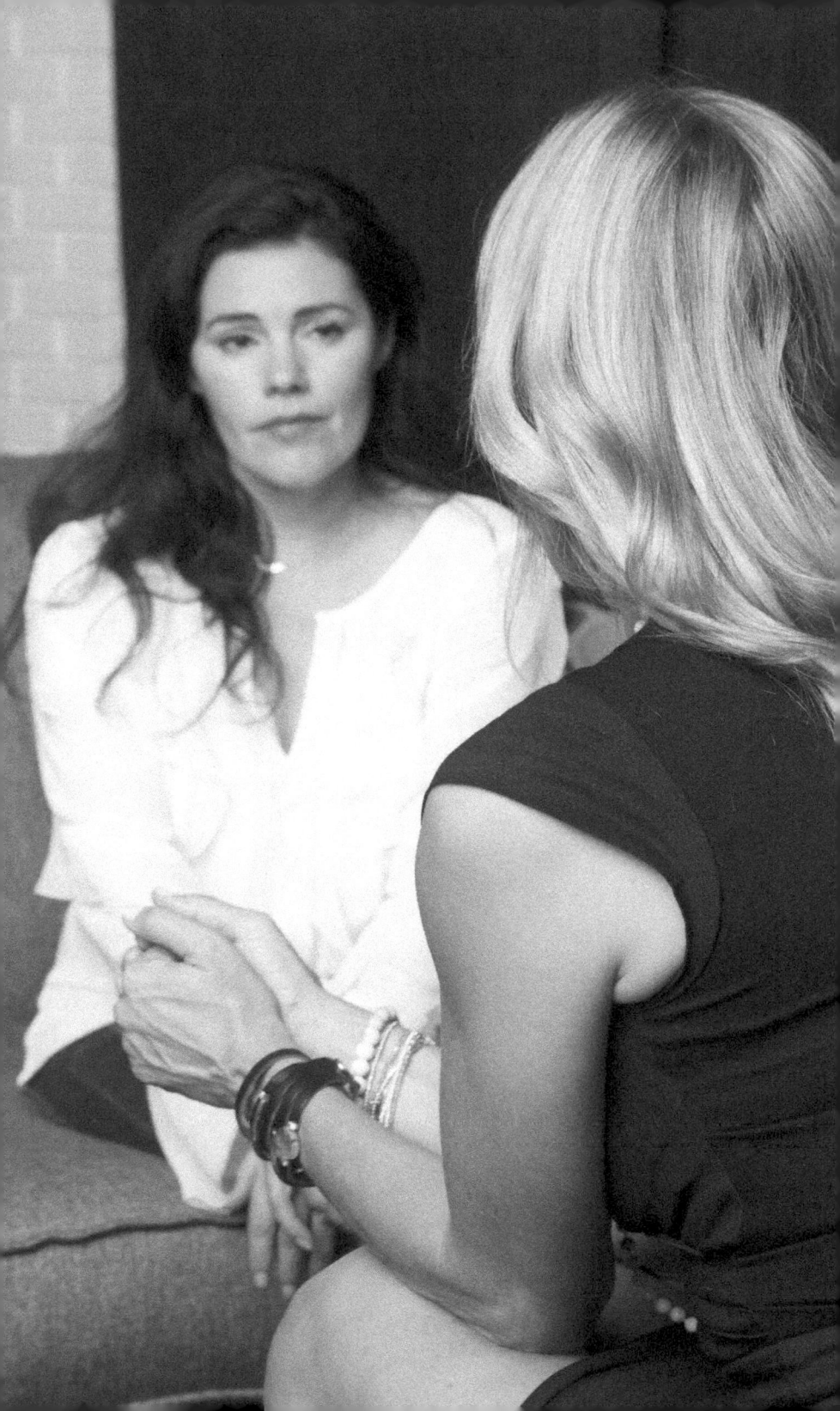

Get it done

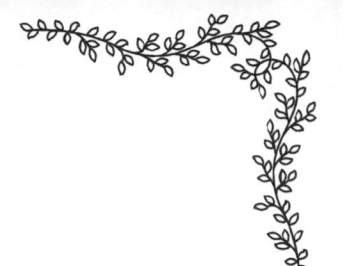

_____

_____

_____

_____

_____

_____

_____

_____

_____

_____

_____

_____

_____

_____

_____

_____

_____

16

Give Without Expectation

When we give freely, we always get something back, even when we're not looking for it. That's the way life works. Giving has little to do with the receiver.

It doesn't matter whether the people we're giving to are giving back to us. In fact, they might not even be grateful receivers, but we always get something in return. Maybe it's the good feeling that comes from sharing, or the satisfaction of knowing we've made someone happy. It might be self-respect or confidence.

Can I say that everything changes when we start expecting to get something back? See, that's not really giving. It's a form of manipulation. Giving freely means the receiver doesn't owe us anything. Not even a thank you.

Give, and then forget you gave. There's no "I paid for lunch last time, so it's your turn to pay" assumption. If the person offers, be a grateful receiver, but freely giving means you're not offended when they don't.

If you give money to someone who needs it, unless you both agree it's a loan, give and then forget you gave it.

Here are a few other ways you can give to others.

- *Let someone talk, tell a story, or share without feeling you have to have a turn to talk. LISTEN.*
- *Be transparent when you know it might be of value to someone. Do it without the expectation that they will necessarily be as open with you.*
- *Make a meal or bake something for someone who could use a kind gesture.*
- *Let someone go ahead of you in line at the market. Even if they have more stuff.*
- *Tell someone how you feel about them. You may think the person knows they are loved, and they might, but think about how good it feels to hear it.*
- *Resist being a know-it-all, even when you know something about a topic being discussed. Let someone teach you something.*
- *Accept a gift from someone without judging it. Even if the person gives you something you don't like or want, show your gratitude for the giving.*

Hey! Want to give big? APOLOGIZE when you've made a mistake or done something to offend. This is hard for some people who feel their actions somehow mean something about them. They don't.

We ALL make mistakes. Apologizing doesn't mean you take responsibility for the other person's reaction. We are all responsible for our own feelings. When you apologize, you're showing empathy. You're letting the other person know you care about how they feel.

GIVE ONLY WHEN YOU MEAN IT

There are so many ways we can give. But a gift is only a gift if we are being genuine. Give only when you want to and not when it's appropriate or expected. Be real!

This includes receiving compliments. Be gracious without feeling you have to return the compliment. Remember, true giving is done without expectation of anything in return. I love the idea of thanking someone for being patient if you arrive late. It sets a different tone than apologizing. Saying thank you, and meaning it, is a gift in itself.

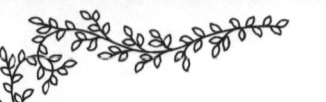

Get it done

_____

_____

_____

_____

_____

_____

_____

_____

_____

_____

_____

_____

_____

_____

_____

_____

Rest and Relaxation

Did you ever wake up on a Saturday and hit the snooze bar instead going for that early morning run you had planned on?

Many of us want to maintain an aggressive exercise routine—particularly when we're seeing results, as in "Hey, have you lost weight?" or "Boy, you're looking great!" But let's face it; sometimes fatigue just catches up with us.

Too much exercise can lead to injuries, exhaustion, and depression according to WebMD, an online resource that offers information on managing our health. Those of us who can't seem to start the day without an intense cardio workout at the gym or a 5-mile run could actually be classified as "exercise addicts," although we might not realize it.

If you're beginning to lose your motivation to go to the gym, it might be time to take a break. And if the exercise routines you normally do without much thought suddenly seem arduous...well, that's another indication that you're probably overdoing it.

Recent research has debunked the notion that late-night workouts can interfere with your sleep patterns. But extreme night sessions can cause insomnia.

The point is, you might need some downtime, whether it's waking up late on a Saturday morning and checking out the local yard sales or stopping off to get a healthy snack on the way home from work. Occasionally you may need to get away from the crazy fitness routine you've established for yourself.

And can I tell you something? It pays off! It's been proven that getting enough rest gives you more energy, enhances your immune system, reduces your blood pressure, and increases your problem-solving abilities. So the time you spend away from those grueling workouts or early morning jogs around the neighborhood might actually benefit your chess game...or not.

If you have trouble getting to sleep, there are a few things you can do that will help. First of all, try to avoid taking naps during the day, and avoid drinks with caffeine or alcohol within six hours of going to bed. Make sure your bedroom is a comfy sleeping environment—not too hot, too cold, or too noisy.

Essential oils can be soothing sleep aids. Make them a part of your bedtime ritual. You'll find your favorites when you experiment. For instance, lavender is calming and helps soothe tension. Bergamot is great for relaxation and can quiet your mind before sleep. Roman chamomile is also a popular oil, and any of the three can be diffused to promote a restful sleep.

By the way, I devoted a chapter of this book to essential oils to give you a better understanding of them. It's coming up!

Note: Find out more information about essential oils and how to use them in my book, *A Beginner's Guide to Essential Oils*. Pick it up on Amazon.

Sleep is important, but there are plenty of other ways to get some rest and relaxation. Yoga can be beneficial since it involves stretching, which tends to be relaxing. Or maybe you'd simply like to listen to some of your favorite music. Led Zeppelin, anyone?

You could also take in a movie or go shopping for that new iPhone you've been eyeing. And the best part? You can do all of these things without breaking a sweat! Hey, no one ever said life couldn't include some fun.

So the next time that alarm goes off on a Saturday morning, remember—you always have the option of hitting the snooze bar. This time it's okay, really!

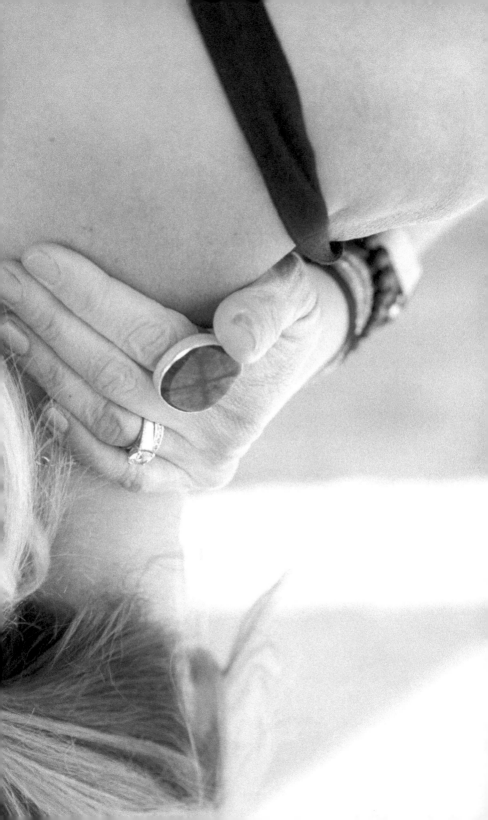

Get it done

_____

_____

_____

_____

_____

_____

_____

_____

_____

_____

_____

_____

_____

_____

_____

_____

_____

_____

_____

_____

_____

18

Eat to Live

Instead of Living to Eat

You are what you eat, right? Well, it's a little more complicated than that, but what you eat definitely affects your quality of life. In the worst-case scenario, what you eat can make you sick.

You can also heal your life with food.

Pay close attention to what you put into your body because it impacts everything: how you feel, think, and live. There's a lot of evidence to support this. If you want to *get it done*, whatever it is, begin with a healthy diet.

Certain foods cause weight gain and water retention. Hormones also have a lot to do with weight management. If you want to lose weight, you have to balance your hormones and regulate the release of insulin in your body. The first place to start is to get off the wheat and sugars!

Come On, Really—How Important Is Diet?

I am vegan. At one point I ate a 100% raw diet. The only reason I am not still exclusively eating raw is I found it too tedious to maintain. But I do enjoy a number of raw foods, and juicing is a huge part of my diet.

Am I saying being vegetarian has no value and carnivores are on a path to destruction? I won't go that far (although I'd like to). But I will say there's plenty of proof of the effects of diet on health.

EATING TO...SLEEP?

You don't have to eat vegan to benefit from a good breakfast. Eat healthy first thing in the morning and you'll sleep better at night. Avoid spicy foods and junk food at night.

A hearty breakfast or lunch is better than stuffing yourself at dinner. Make a habit of eating light in the latter part of the day. Heavy meals increase your risk of indigestion, and drinking a lot after 7 p.m. means you're likely to spend half the night in the bathroom.

If you suffer from insomnia, a light dinner or snack about two hours before bed can actually help you sleep better. Operative word: light.

GLUTEN INTOLERANCE

You might be thinking that the popularity of gluten-free food items is in response to a fad; kind of like he Atkins Diet and others in the past. But if you're gluten-intolerant, you know it is not.

A diet low in gluten is definitely healthier. But it's transforming the lives of people who have never known what it was like to be without stomach pains and other symptoms associated with gluten intolerance.

I'm not talking about a little tummy ache after dinner, either. Digestive symptoms such as excruciating abdominal pain, bloating, and diarrhea are bad enough. Most also suffer from gluten-induced anxiety, depression, headaches, and exhaustion. Removing gluten from their diets has been nothing less than a miracle.

It used to be if you wanted to buy gluten-free food items, you had to go a specialty store. Not anymore! Gluten-free foods are becoming widely available in most mainstream supermarkets. There are also gluten-free choices on restaurant menus.

DIABETES: THE SILENT KILLER

How do you know if you have diabetes? The signs can be subtle, and you might not notice until it's too late. This is especially true for Type 2 diabetes. Below are common symptoms to pay attention to, just in case....

If you're experiencing any of these, check with your doctor.

- *You're hungrier and more tired than usual*
- *Need to pee more often than usual*
- *Dry mouth*
- *Itchy skin (might signal dehydration)*
- *Blurred vision*

Regardless of how you choose to eat, changing your habits can take some time. It can be challenging to turn away from foods you love even though you know they aren't good for you.

Ask a sugar addict. You might be able to do it cold turkey, or it can take time. The point is, you're making changes, and that's better than allowing denial to keep intoxicating you.

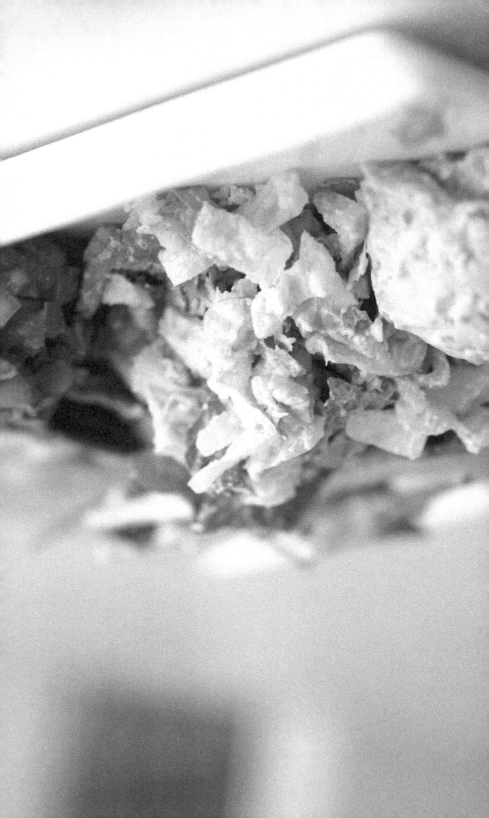

Get it done

_____

_____

_____

_____

_____

_____

_____

_____

_____

_____

_____

_____

_____

_____

_____

_____

19

Release Toxins

Cleanse and Then Keep It Clean

Discussing toxins is a bigger discussion than what's in your FOOD. But food is a major part of this discussion and is something you need to think seriously about. Some of the food you eat is not even real. You might as well be gnawing on plastic.

In the US, the typical American diet is serving up a death sentence.

Processed, unhealthy foods can really do a number on your body.

Do you feel fatigued? Low energy? You might chalk it up to not sleeping well, but it's more likely that you're not eating well.

Listen to your body! It will usually tell you when something's not right. The signs can be subtle, like bad breath. Bacteria in your mouth can cause bad breath, but persistent bad breath can also indicate that your liver and/or kidneys are having trouble filtering toxins out of your bloodstream.

It's easy to inadvertently consume toxins when they're in our food and drinks. Hydrogenated oil and MSG are a couple of obvious toxins, but there's something far worse—artificial sweeteners, such as Aspartame and Sucralose. They're hazardous to your health. Avoid them.

It might seem super hard at first, but one of the most important steps you can take is to start eating foods that are natural instead of processed. Processed foods contain toxins, and as you phase them out, you'll probably start feeling a lot better—and it won't take long.

When you detoxify, your body returns to its natural state—one without man-made chemicals and poisons floating around causing damage. Go organic and eat dark, leafy greens, dark berries, and other foods that are high in antioxidants, which do battle with free radicals; free radicals are particles that travel around the body potentially damaging tissues with which they come into contact.

Fabric and carpet treatments contain tons of hazardous chemicals. So do air fresheners and scented candles. When you combine these household items with cleaning products, you've got a potentially nasty mix of toxins. You can inadvertently consume them when they become airborne and land on plates, food, or anywhere else.

Still, you can eat all the tofu and raw gritty kale you want, but if your life is toxic, your sacrifices will have very little value. A major part of living healthy is removing toxicity from your life. It's your job, and you're the only one who can do it.

Toxic Relationships

Toxicity shows up in a couple of ways; one thing that tends to slip under the radar is an addiction to toxic relationships. Toxic relationships can hurt you in so many ways, and unfortunately they aren't always easy to spot, because you can't put all the blame on one person. It always takes two. Healthy people aren't in toxic relationships unless they participate in them.

Are you in a toxic relationship? Just because you're a badass doesn't mean you have to tough it out.

Chances are if one of your relationships is toxic, others might be, too. How do you know if a relationship is toxic? Here are a few signs.

FEARING A PARTNER'S EMOTIONAL REACTIONS

Your partner doesn't have to grab you by the throat or yell at you to be physically or verbally abusive. All it takes is for you to fear their emotional reactions. If you find yourself having to bite your tongue because you're afraid of how your partner may react to your opinion, you may be in a toxic relationship.

COMPROMISE? WHAT'S COMPROMISE?

It's a sign of trouble when the give-and-take in your relationship means you always give and your partner always takes. Whether the person is a romantic partner or a friend, all healthy relationships need some sort of compromise to keep both parties happy. One person shouldn't win every time.

PASSIVE-AGGRESSIVE PATTERNS

Sometimes passive-aggressive behavior is worse than straight-out aggression. It's a really unhealthy way of expressing anger. When someone is being passive-aggressive, they may find subtle ways to irritate you. Passive-aggressive communication usually results in bigger fights and arguments. If there's a communication breakdown, find ways to either address it or reassess whether you should be together at all.

PROJECTING EMOTIONS

When you project your emotions onto someone, you're essentially blaming them for the way you feel. The other person is not the cause of your pain. If you're unhappy, ask for what you want. If you don't get it and you're unwilling to compromise (which is okay), then leave.

Get it done

_____

_____

_____

_____

_____

_____

_____

_____

_____

_____

_____

_____

_____

_____

_____

_____

_____

_____

_____

_____

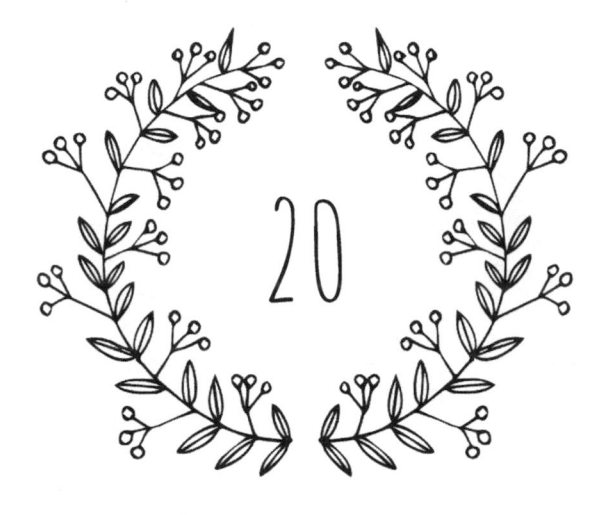

20

Exercise

Move Your Body Every Day

Let's get this straight. Contrary to popular belief, I DO NOT love to work out. I know it's good for me, and so I suck it up and do it religiously. It might be tough getting started, but it gets easier as I go, and it feels so good to breathe!

I see the benefits of exercise in so many ways: more energy and confidence, strength, fitting better in my jeans— meaning I don't have to unbutton them when I sit down. So I suck it up and do it diligently most days of the week.

When I travel, that's my excuse to rest. I used to be super neurotic when I was training as an elite athlete. I woke up at 5 a.m. to get a run in before an early morning flight. Ha! Not any more.

Now I recognize the idea of *balance*, and I use my travel days as rest days. Good thing I travel a lot. That means I get at least one to three days off a week. Sometimes seven days in a row!

Oh, and now that I purposefully attend fitness *classes*, I don't pretend I'm working out when I'm really looking at my phone. I stuff that celly in my bag or a locker. People can survive without me for 45 minutes.

And as far as the 20-minute workout—I have DEFINITELY noted a difference in my fitness when I do HIIT (high intensity interval training) for shorter periods of time rather than being a cardio junkie for an hour or more. Sure, I feel like I'm going to throw up after, but I grab a juice or smoothie and I'm fine. Plus I go to sleep earlier because it exhausts me. No kidding—just those 20–25 minutes.

There are peeps who sit around watching hours of TV every day and only exercise walking back and forth from the refrigerator.

Does the idea of exercise make YOU tired? Come on! Get up and get going. And while you're at it, get up early.

Our bodies are made to move. When you exercise, you don't just burn calories and fat. Other positive changes are taking place throughout your body. Your mood is altered in a positive way, for one.

Psychologists agree that exercise helps combat depression and anxiety. A study conducted at Penn State University found that people who exercised were generally happier on the days they worked out than those who didn't. The study also found that the harder the workout, the happier the people became. Who can't use a little more HAPPY in their life?

Okay, so exercise certainly isn't a cure-all for everything, but it will help with your quality of life, especially if you do it regularly. Find

something you enjoy—a sport, a daily Pilates routine, or running—and then do it.

Everyone starts somewhere, right? Some peeps can jog for half an hour with little difficulty, while others find a 30-minute walk more fun. No matter what you choose to do, if you want to start a routine or get into better shape, set specific, realistic goals. Just like you do with everything else, break your goals down into daily steps.

For example, if your goal is to jog for 30 minutes without stopping and you've been a couch potato for 15 years or more, start wherever you feel comfortable—even if it's five minutes. No kidding. There's value in every step you take toward your goal.

Increase the length of time you run every day by 5-30 seconds until you reach your final goal of 30 minutes. Who knows, you may exceed it. In fact, you probably will.

Meeting and beating your exercise goals will jazz up your self-confidence to tackle more complicated goals in other areas.

Boost Your Energy

We all feel low energy once in a while. If you have a lot of responsibilities that make for long days, it can be worse. This may not make sense at first, but exercising when you're feeling low energy can actually leave you with more energy than when you started. Seriously! Even walking can help you feel more alert, awake, and ready for anything that comes your way.

You don't need to sweat it out with heavy lifting or vigorous sprinting. A 20-minute walk is enough to get your blood pumping and clear your head. Try it next time stress gets the best of you.

REDUCE YOUR RISK OF CARDIOVASCULAR DISEASE

You know, cardiovascular disease is the number one cause of death for people in the US. It's said to be responsible for one out of four deaths! Exercise will not only change your life, it could prolong your life. Your heart is a muscle, and like other muscles in your body, when you exercise it, it gets stronger.

Studies have shown that cardio is just as effective as medications in preventing heart disease. In 2012 a study of 650,000 people found that an hour and a half of moderate exercise every week increases your lifespan by 3.4 years.

We could all use a little extra time to enjoy life! Life is beautiful. Exercise can help you keep creating memories and be there for yourself and loved ones. It's worth the effort. Get started!

Along with exercise, I'm a yoga buff. There are tons of benefits.

Check it out in the next chapter.

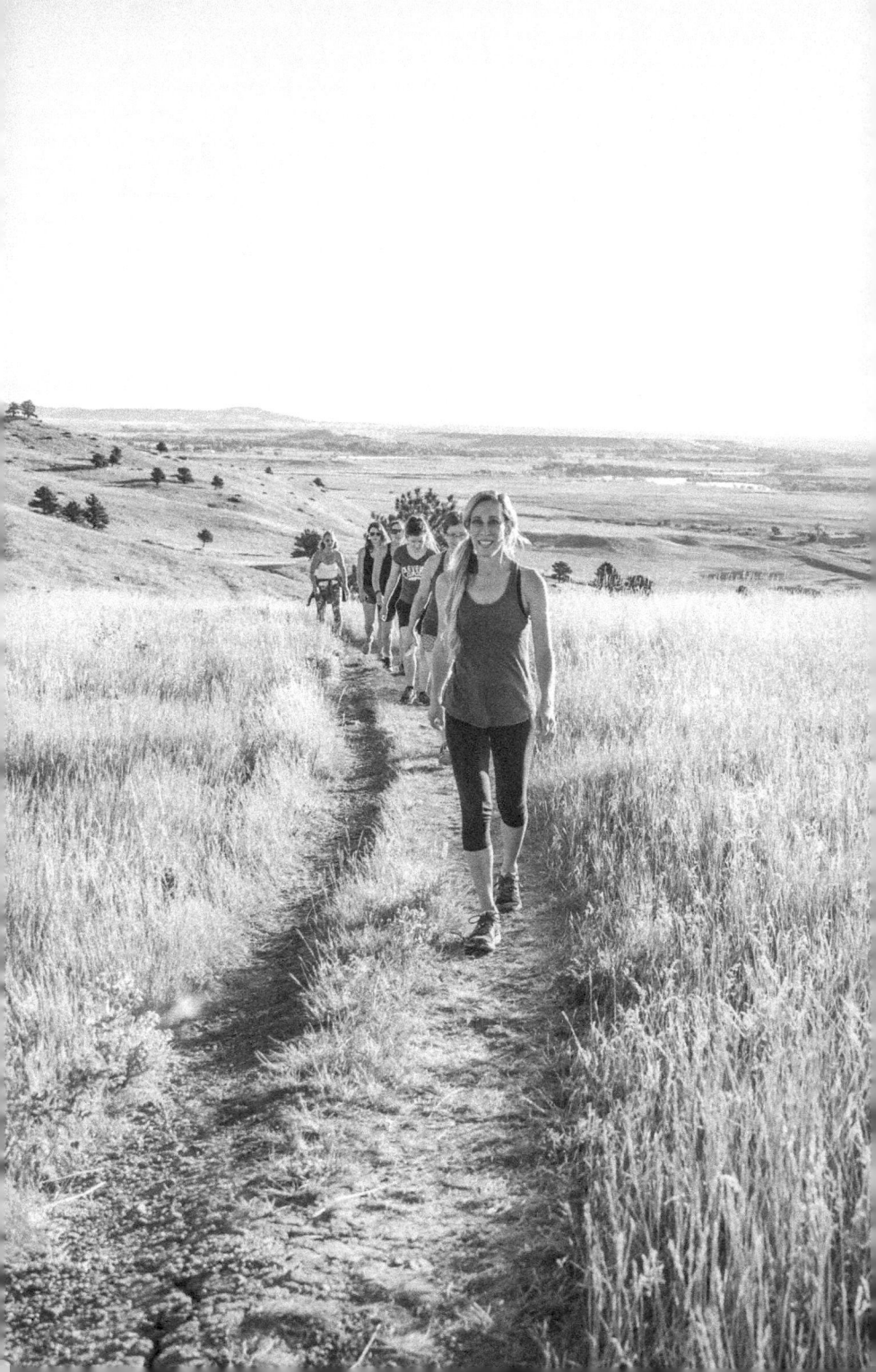

Get it done

_____

_____

_____

_____

_____

_____

_____

_____

_____

_____

_____

_____

_____

_____

_____

_____

_____

_____

_____

_____

Practice Yoga

So, yoga...

Whether you're into it or not, I have a few things to say about yoga. It's one of my passions—I taught yoga for 15 years. We're talking balance here, and this is one of the most important chapters in this book—even for that inner boss of yours. So grab a juice and stick with me for a couple of pages, okay?

If you're already dabbling in yoga, you already know what I'm about to say. And if you're just getting started, I want you to know you don't have to work up to the benefits of yoga. Even beginners feel the joy and balance immediately. In fact, you don't have to be super bendy to practice yoga. The stiffer you are, the more progress you make.

But there are a few challenges you may have to get through to get the full benefit.

One is the vocabulary.

The traditional language of yoga is Sanskrit. It's not like French or Spanish where you can pretty much sound out the words. Terms like *asana* and *prana* are not so bad, but Sanskrit words such as *pashchimottan asana* might tangle your tongue. Do you have to speak Sanskrit to do yoga? No, but if you're going all in, it's important to understand the terminology.

Yoga Classes

You might think you need to live in a big city to find a yoga class nearby. Not true! You can live in the woods a mile away from a town with a population of 4,000 and usually still find a yoga class. Google "yoga classes" in your area or look at ads in health publications. You can also practice yoga at home by yourself if you can put together a series of techniques or pop in a DVD class. Even YouTube.com can support your yoga practice!

You don't have to be thin to practice yoga. Even if you're not at your most ideal body weight, you can still get on board with this. Some of the postures can be challenging at first, but nobody expects you to be perfect.

The best way to learn yoga is to attend a class, or if you can afford it, private instruction. The positions can be awkward at first. Don't worry, it's not you.

Be patient with yourself. Your body needs to be flexible with specific movements it may never have experienced.

Some positions require you to balance on one foot, and in the beginning, it might be helpful to practice next to a wall to steady yourself. Balance comes with practice.

It's important to have instruction when you're starting out; especially just to be sure you're getting the postures down correctly.

Trust me, it's better to learn yoga correctly the first time than to have to unlearn incorrect patterns and then repattern.

Yoga is not just a physical activity. It will help you balance your life because it's a body-mind-spirit practice. The following tips will be helpful:

YOUR YOGA SPACE

Make a space in your home or outside where you do your yoga routine. Even when you're not doing yoga, you will feel relaxed and balanced anywhere near it.

JOURNAL YOUR THOUGHTS

A spiral-bound practice journal or perfect-bound journal work in the same way. Both will track your progress and evolution through yoga. Another thing you can use it for is to compile a list of postures.

INVEST IN A STICKY MAT

So if you're thinking you can do yoga without a mat, you're right. But if you want to do it well, a yoga mat or sticky mat will make a world of difference. If you're not sure, borrow one and see for yourself.

Whether you're using your own or sharing one with a friend, remember to keep your sticky mat clean. They get super gross! Spray it down with melaleuca oil (tea tree oil) often. It works great. In the next chapter I'll tell you more about essential oils, including about how they saved my life.

YOGA FOR WEIGHT LOSS?

Sounds crazy, right? It surely doesn't seem that you burn a lot of calories. How can a slow, relaxed program like yoga help with weight loss?

Along with movement, doing yoga will help you think in different ways. When you feel better—which you will—you'll be more clear and focused. As your thinking changes, so will your actions. If you've been overeating, you'll bring your diet into balance. Exercise will begin to feel good, and you'll be motivated instead of exhausted at the thought!

The best thing about yoga is that it works on all of you!
Learn how to move and how to think in new ways. You'll
also learn how to breathe.

BALANCE THROUGH BREATHING

Okay, so YOU may be evolving, but what do you do if
your environment stays the same? Life can be chaotic. All
the more reason to learn how to cope! One way to bring
balance into your life through yoga is breathing.

Breathing is in itself a powerful tool for managing stress
and tension. Along with breathing being super valuable in
stressful situations, teach yourself how to breathe regularly
even when the waters are calm. Even a few minutes once
or twice a day can make a HUGE difference.

Yoga, breathing, and meditation work together. Each is
related to the other and each has its own set of benefits.
Once you get past that voice in your head that says you
can't do it or you don't have time, you'll be on your way
to finding balance no matter where you are.

Get it done

_____

_____

_____

_____

_____

_____

_____

_____

_____

_____

_____

_____

_____

_____

_____

_____

_____

_____

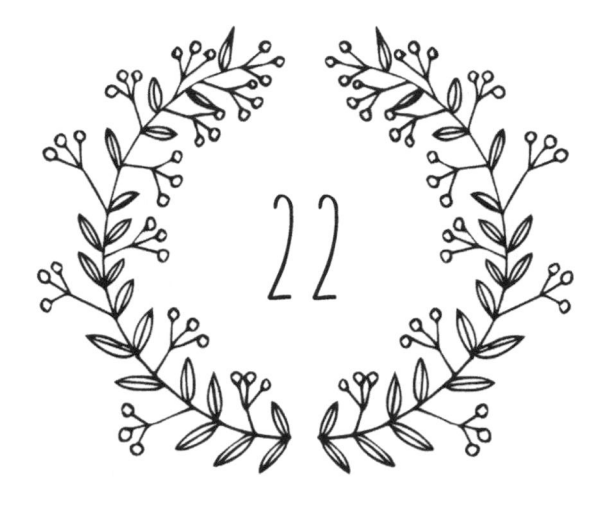

Essential Oils

To Know Them Is to Love Them

I'm not going to sugarcoat this. It's true that essential oils saved my life.

Several years ago, I was losing steam fast. My body was responding to my lifestyle and mental health, neither of which were very healthy. In fact, I was on the fast track to the grave, and my foot was on the gas.

I've told you about my career as an attorney—how I got there and why I walked away. But I haven't told you this part of my story.

Physically, I was a mess. I was suffering from poor digestion and hardly eating because of it. I almost never felt well. Add this to my emotional distress, and it didn't seem like there was much to live for.

One day a realization hit me like a slap in the face. I was at a crossroads. I needed to take an honest look at my life and where I was headed, and then STOP, own up to my choices, and turn and walk in another direction.

Obviously I chose to take this on. I wouldn't have written this book if I hadn't. Honestly, I wouldn't be here today.

It took a lot of courage to make new choices, but you know what? I was ready to make them, and I am so grateful to my inner boss—the part of me that picked me up and set me on my current path.

Along the way, I discovered essential oils. They not only helped support a healthy immune system but also aided in transforming my mental and emotional life.

WHAT ARE ESSENTIAL OILS?

Essential oils are naturally occurring compounds found in flowers and plants. They also come from tree bark, seeds, roots, and other parts of plants besides flowers. The scents you smell from plants come from essential oils. Over 3,000 essential oils have been identified. My favorites are the citrus oils.

In addition to essential oils as useful parts of a lifestyle that proactively boosts your immune and digestive systems, helps balance your hormones, and keeps you from freaking out, essential oils can be used in beauty treatments and cooking. There are also recipes that combine different oils for specific purposes.

Essential oils are gifts from the earth. Using them has changed my life in so many ways. By learning about their true potential, I discovered my own.

My Relationship with Essential Oils

I actually started promoting essential oils before I discovered personal health benefits. And then once I experienced the changes that came from using essential oils, I felt compelled to share them with others, and so I taught others about how to use them to better their quality of life.

Keep in mind, back then I had nothing to invest in my business except me. Yeah, that happens when you walk away from a 6-figure annual income. So there I was with no skills, no network, and nothing but a desire to help others who wanted the same things I did. So I stepped onto the first rung of the ladder and began my climb.

Even though money is not first on my list of what is important, I believe it's more than okay to earn money—to prosper doing something you love. So I worked at building my business. Yeah, it was hard work and it took time, but at the same time, essential oils sell themselves.

Today I have a super successful business promoting healthy living and the use of essential oils. I believe they're part of a holistic regimen that includes a healthy diet and exercise—among other things, of course.

Anyone who knows me will tell you essential oils are a big part of my life. I use them both to help me relax and to energize me. I use oils so I don't miss out on the mornings when it's my turn to get everyone out of the house so I can get to my workout class on time.

Truth? You want to know what I love most about my oils? They allow me to navigate the massive amount of chaos going on around me. I carry as many as I can fit in my purse and pack them when I travel. Everyone in my family, all the way down to my seven-year-old daughter, uses oils.

Remember that everything works together—oils, diet, exercise, meditation—all of it—to help you be well and get it done.

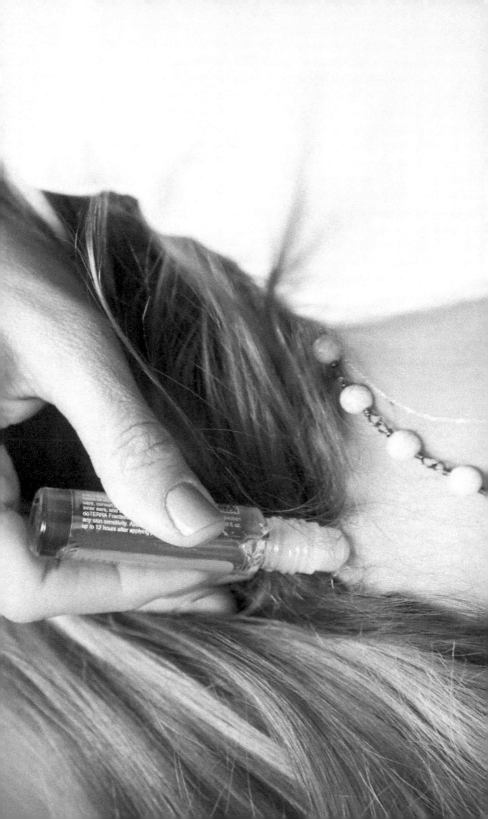

Get it done

_____

_____

_____

_____

_____

_____

_____

_____

_____

_____

_____

_____

_____

_____

_____

_____

_____

_____

23

Prayer and Meditation

We are living in a world of stress, no doubt about it.

And it's coming at us from every direction. When we watch the evening news or check the news reports on our smart phones, we're inundated with it. If it's not a terrorist attack, it's a police shooting...or maybe a multi-car pileup.

And that's just the stuff going on around us. We also have stress in our personal lives—from the stress of worrying about paying bills and making our monthly mortgage payments to stress related to family members or friends who are dealing with serious illness.

Prayer and meditation—even quiet reflection—can help. Dealing with these kinds of stresses is far easier if you can get outside yourself—or more accurately, *inside* yourself— and kick all of those worries to the curb.

Meditation is a great way to calm your nerves and get in touch with the super powerful potential of your unconscious mind. It can break down barriers and free you to better handle the challenges that end up on your doorstep.

This doesn't have to be a big production. Sometimes taking five or ten minutes off the grid and focusing on the inner you can take you to a whole different place. If you do this regularly, you'll soon find that you're more relaxed and more able to achieve your goals in life.

A great thing about meditation is you don't have to be sitting still or lying down when you do it. Just don't do it while you're driving!

You could be walking along your favorite hiking path when you take yourself to that special place, or you could even do it while you're cleaning the bathroom.

Meditation can be a kind of self-guided imagery that involves progressive relaxation and creative visualization—and ultimately, stress relief. Some people focus on a word or image.

Remember that body, mind, and spirit are all connected. Meditation can provide lots of physiological benefits, such as lowering your oxygen consumption, decreasing your respiratory rate, increasing blood flow, increasing exercise tolerance, and decreasing muscle tension.

And let's not forget prayer. Nothing in life can be more personal—or more rewarding—than having open communication with God. *The Christian Post* says you should "never underestimate the power of prayer."

Prayer produces a feeling of peacefulness. It eliminates worry and anxiety and can give you energy. It also shields you from discouragement. And let's face it; there are plenty of things going on around us to be discouraged about. But by connecting with your inner consciousness, either through meditation or prayer, you open doors that would otherwise remain shut.

It's all about self-motivation.

I personally enjoy moving meditation, which for me is simply the act of being aware of my body or my breathing while I'm working out, washing the dishes, or even taking a walk.

SELF-HYPNOSIS

Now here's something interesting. You have access to it, 24/7. Self-hypnosis can help you relax anytime, anywhere. As with meditation, you can use guided imagery, progressive relaxation, or creative visualization. Go to a safe place in your mind. Clear negativity, and dissolve stress and tension. Google sample self-inductions or check Youtube. com for videos.

Get it done

_____

_____

_____

_____

_____

_____

_____

_____

_____

_____

_____

_____

_____

_____

_____

_____

24

Learn How to Play

Come On, Make Time for Fun!

Can you remember what it felt like to run outside and stay there until your mom called you home? Remember the buzz you got when you were playing games with the neighborhood kids? Or how about the time you climbed that big tree in the backyard and got your first view of the whole neighborhood around you? It was awesome, wasn't it? Those kinds of childhood memories are etched in the mind.

It makes me smile whenever I see Madeline using her imagination or when I hear the ridiculousness of her stories. It's the best feeling ever. I often laugh out loud.

Why is it as we grow older many of us have less and less time for play? We're so busy paying our bills and worrying about the next project that we develop a kind of tunnel vision. We see what's in front of us—all of those things that need to get done—and we forget to let loose.

Somewhere along the way to adulthood we forgot how to play and what it feels like to do something just for the fun of it. And that's one of the best parts of life. Have you ever gone to a department store with a 5-year-old? If they get anywhere near the toy aisle, their eyes light right up. They let go of your hand and run, right? They run toward their favorite toys and get lost in imagination.

As adults, we often forget how to do that. When we do manage to carve out some leisure time, we're more likely to zone out in front of the TV or computer than engage in real fun like we did when we were kids. It's not too late to get those feelings back.

Play doesn't have to be a tough workout at the gym, although exercise can be playtime. Or the next time you have a weekend morning off, find a hiking trail and trek up into the hills. Call a friend and see a movie. If you have kids, power down your computer and run around outside with them.

Be in the moment. Put the brakes on the mayhem and enjoy some time to yourself.

Why is play important?

It can relieve stress and improve brain function. It can be exhilarating! Play stimulates the mind, and you know what else it can do? It can improve your relationships with others. People who know how to play are fun to hang out with.

Play can also heal relationships when they're on the rocks because of resentments or disagreements. Think about it. It's hard to be angry with someone when you're laughing together and having a good time.

What do you like to do? Play board games? Go on day trips? Take a cruise? Learn something new, or do something you've never done.

Slow down, create, and make space for the unpredictable! Laugh until it hurts.

Whatever you enjoy doing, set some time aside. Balance work with play. AND schedule it so you don't fill the space in your days just with work. Don't allow the stress and commotion of everyday life to be your only focus.

Get dirty and break the rules once in a while.

Take five!

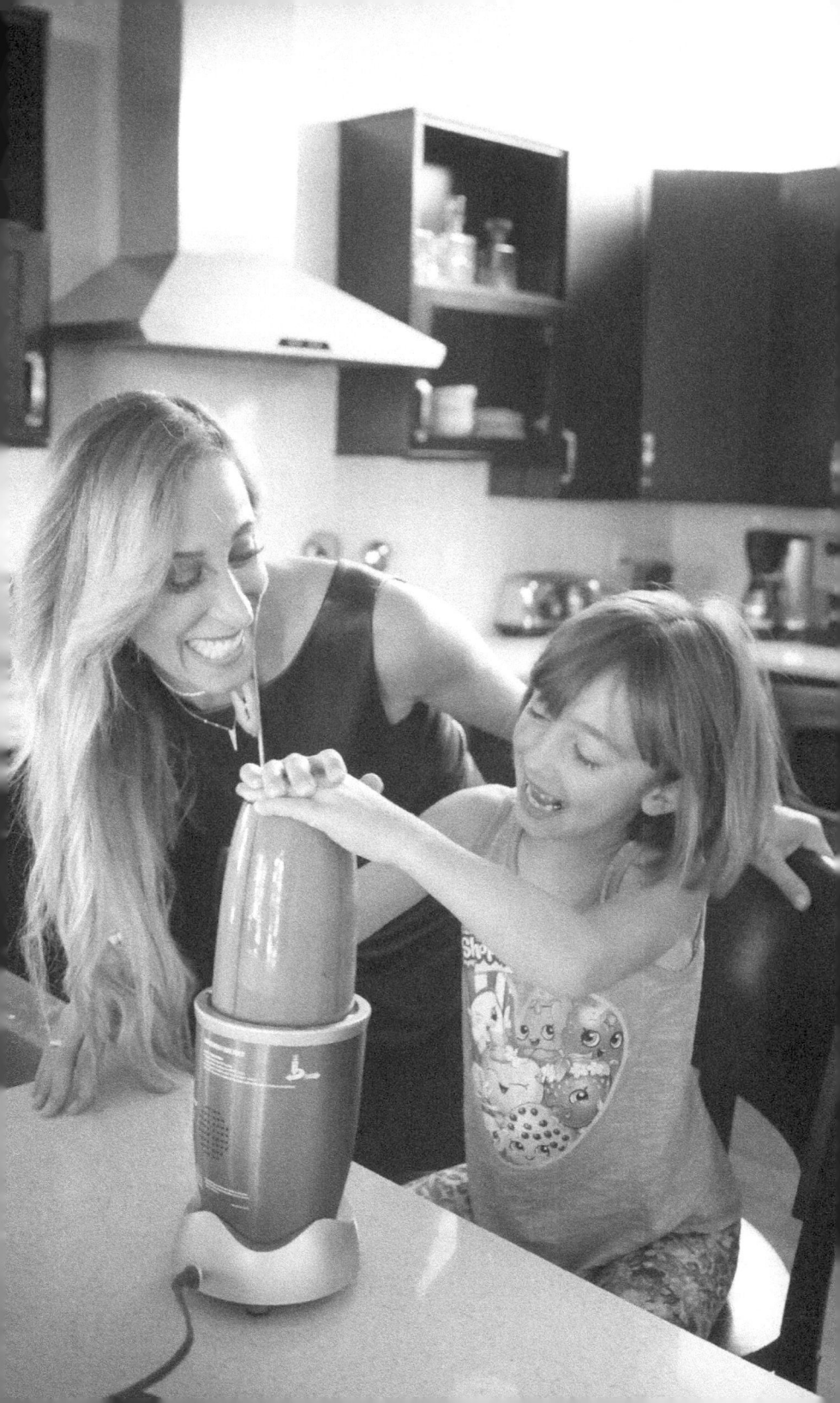

Get it done

_____

_____

_____

_____

_____

_____

_____

_____

_____

_____

_____

_____

_____

_____

_____

_____

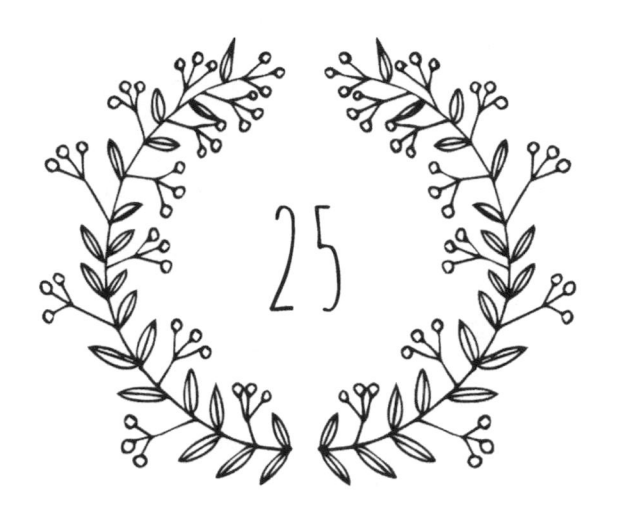

25

Smile Wide and Laugh Out Loud

Few things in life are as easy as a smile, and few things can boost your mood as quickly.

And the neat thing about a smile is that it can come out of nowhere. It could be prompted by a funny joke, a TV comedy show, or maybe something you happen to see during the course of your day, like a toddler trying to eat ice cream for the first time or a puppy running around the yard. Regardless of what prompts it, a smile simply makes you feel better.

If you're having a bad day at work, a funny remark from a coworker can quickly turn things around. But there are also real medical benefits, too. A smile can help you manage stress and anxiety by releasing endorphins. Endorphins are the same chemicals you get from working out or running. So in essence, you could get a runner's high without even lacing up your shoes!

A smile also makes you more attractive to others. Have you ever walked into a store and seen someone with a scowl on their face—someone who looks like they just drank some spoiled milk? Yikes! Unfortunately, some people are like that all the time. They may not be aware of it, but they walk around looking like they don't want ANYONE to speak to them. You don't want to be that person!

You'll be much more approachable if you have a smile on your face. So whether you're at a party with friends or at a nightclub hoping to connect with someone special, having a smile on your face will put you ahead of the game. People are naturally drawn to others who seem to be happy.

And smiles can definitely make a difference at work. You can joke with coworkers during breaks or relieve stress at lunch by shooting hoops. It will strengthen the bond you have with them and also boost your job performance.

A study published by the National Institutes of Health revealed that hospitalized children who were entertained by visitors who told them stories and put on puppet shows ended up smiling and laughing. It also boosted the children's white blood cell counts.

Smiles do a lot more than let the world know you're happy. Heck, they don't even have to be genuine to have some effect. But you can find plenty of things in your life to smile about. Just look around—check out that beautiful sunset at the end of the day or the way the clouds drift by on a warm, sunny afternoon.

If that doesn't prompt a smile, wait until your son or daughter runs up to you and says, "Look Mom, I got an A on my math test!" Or wait until you find out that your income tax refund is going to be nearly double the amount you were expecting. That would be enough to make anyone smile!

So the next time you're in need of a pick-me-up, look around. If you're out driving, pull the friggin' car over and take a peek at the sunset. Wherever or whatever you're driving to can wait an extra five minutes. Watch until the sun sizzles on the horizon. Now that will make you smile.

And don't stop there. Open wide and laugh out loud no matter who's listening!

So, I'm sure you've heard the expression, "Laughter is the best medicine." It's the truth! Unless you have to pee, that is. Then it's a liability. When you get to be a *certain age*, the trick is to cross your legs when you laugh. Know that one?

We laugh for joy—sometimes with uncontrollable laughter and at other times with private snickers only we are aware of. Don't cover your mouth and hold back. Laugh out loud! Trust me, it won't make you less cool.

Laughing out loud can be a super cool fix when diving through the dailies. Dealing with life isn't always like floating on cream puffs. It can also be like skidding downhill on a gravel road—on your bare knees.

Sometimes just getting through the day is a chore. When you're having challenges with your budget, it can be stressful, right? It depends on your outlook! We've all been there.

Look for the silly side, and yes, there's a super silly side to everything. Flipping on the tube and zoning can have its benefits as long as you don't overdo it.

I suspect more than a few people turn on Comedy Central at the end of the day or some other satirical perusal of our collective human condition. At the time of this writing, Saturday Night Live is experiencing the highest ratings it has seen in 20 years.

We often deal with life's trials through laughter. Finding the absurdity in situations can make all the difference to our experience. It's not bad for sanity maintenance, either, especially when we're dealing with chaos.

Life comes with hurdles. Laughter is YOUR pole vault. The more you use it, the better it serves.

OTHER BENEFITS OF LAUGHTER

Laughter just plain makes you feel better, doesn't it? I love to laugh. A good laugh releases endorphins and exercises the stomach muscles. It creates warm spaces between others and us.

You may have heard crying helps release toxins from the body? Well, laughter serves the same purpose!

Laughing at life is pretty much required if you want to keep moving past barriers—including those you put in place yourself. There's even proof that laughter boosts your immune system by increasing the number of antibody-producing T cells. This means a good chuckle can help you fight colds and flu.

Optimistic people live longer than pessimists. There have been some pretty cool comedians who proved this themselves, like Bob Hope, who lived to be over 100 years old and traveled the world on USO tours bringing laughter to stressed-out service people. And George Burns was another guy who lived laughter and made it to 100 years old. Norman Cousins cured himself from cancer with laughter and went on to impact the world with his work.

The most chaotic and stressful moments are when laughter is most important. It'll change your brain chemistry. And laughter is contagious. When you laugh out loud, it makes others want to laugh too. In giving and sharing laughter, everybody benefits.

Some people can't help laughing. They find everything funny—even when it's really not. There are also folks who are so crazy serious they have trouble finding their funny bone. Where do you fall on the spectrum?

Lighten up! There are Laughter Therapy classes, and there is even Laughter Yoga to help if you need a nudge.

Laughter will elevate your mood and decrease stress and anxiety. Get out of your comfort zone, even when your head is wrapped around a big project. Laughing out loud will put light back in the room.

Laughter helps you lose weight. There. Got your attention, didn't I?

Seriously, it's really good exercise. Laughter raises your heart rate and speeds up your metabolism.

If you laugh on a regular basis, you can lower your blood pressure. When you first start to laugh, your blood pressure goes up, but after a good laugh, it decreases to levels on the low side of normal.

A big belly laugh is a good thing! Open wide and let it out.

Research shows 15 minutes of laughter a day is as important as 30 minutes of exercise a day. It helps you stay healthy, and if you're sick, it helps you feel better.

Get it done

_____

_____

_____

_____

_____

_____

_____

_____

_____

_____

_____

_____

_____

_____

_____

_____

_____

_____

_____

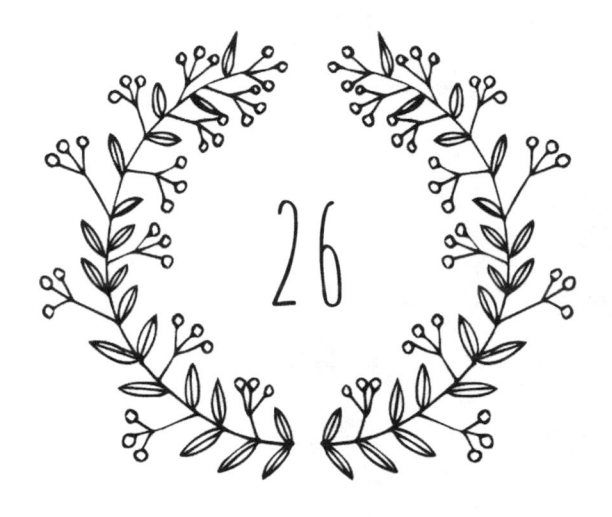

Give Thanks

Saying "thank you" is not going to cramp your style. In fact, saying "thank you" will win more points with people who say or do things for you. Thank yourself once in a while, too.

Here's a great practice to cultivate: express gratitude the moment you open your eyes in the morning. Create your day in your mind by listing off everything you're grateful for in advance of getting it. Be grateful for the good and the bad, knowing it's all leading you somewhere.

It's scientifically proven that gratitude opens the door to building relationships. Saying "thank you" is more than good manners, it also helps you express appreciation to family and friends.

A study published in 2014 found that *thanking a new acquaintance* makes them more likely to want to continue a relationship with you. Acknowledging other people's gestures can lead to new opportunities for both of you. Thank people who comment on your social media. Acknowledgment goes a long way.

What about thanking yourself? Be grateful for your body and your good health. Grateful people are also more likely to take care of their health. Valuing life will make you want to exercise more often, and you'll be more likely to have regular check-ups.

Gratitude reduces emotional toxicity. Things like envy and resentment will be reduced to little to nothing if you are grateful for what you have. Citing the things you're grateful for will prompt you to pay attention, and you'll notice more for which to be grateful. This is a super effective way to soothe depression. It also helps you sleep more soundly.

Cultivate gratitude. Rather than complain about the things you think you deserve, focus on all that you *have*. Develop an attitude of gratitude. It's really one of the simplest ways to breed happiness and satisfaction in your life. Your life doesn't have to change for you to be grateful, but your life WILL change because of it.

Get it done

_____

_____

_____

_____

_____

_____

_____

_____

_____

_____

_____

_____

_____

_____

_____

_____

_____

_____

27

Hug, Squeeze, and Embrace

When you were little and you fell down and scraped your knee, who came running to your rescue? Who wrapped her arms around you and held you close? Probably your mom, or someone else who loved you very much. Remember how you felt? The world suddenly seemed better, didn't it?

No matter what your circumstances, a simple hug can melt pain away. It reinforces how much you are loved, and when you're the one doing the hugging, it shows you how much you love.

But it goes deeper than that. Hugging offers more than temporary immediate comfort. Yep, research has shown when someone hugs you, it causes your muscles to relax. It can also relieve tension that may have built up from a chaotic day—traffic congestion, the argument you had with that crazy rude guy at the market, or just about any other blackboard scratching annoyance you can imagine.

Ever heard of dopamine? It's one of four chemicals in the brain that influence our sense of happiness. Low dopamine levels are often found in people with Parkinson's disease, and low dopamine levels can also lead to depression.

Well, guess what? Hugging boosts the production of dopamine. So the next time someone you care about is feeling down, give him or her a hug.

Hugs are also a natural pain reliever. When someone wraps their arms around you, it releases endorphins, those all-purpose chemicals that boost happiness. That hug you shared will actually block pain pathways and increase circulation.

A HUG CAN SAVE A LIFE

Do you or does someone you know suffer from high blood pressure? It's one of the main risk factors for heart disease. Hugs to the rescue! Studies have shown that hugging lowers blood pressure and can reduce the risk of heart disease.

You can benefit from a few squishy hugs on a Saturday night while you're watching a movie with your love. Wash away the day's worries and stress.

Hugs also increase feelings of trust. A hug is free. It feels great and actually has healing properties. So I guess it turns out there's some truth to that saying, *"The best things in life are free."*

Get it done

_____

_____

_____

_____

_____

_____

_____

_____

_____

_____

_____

_____

_____

_____

_____

_____

_____

_____

_____

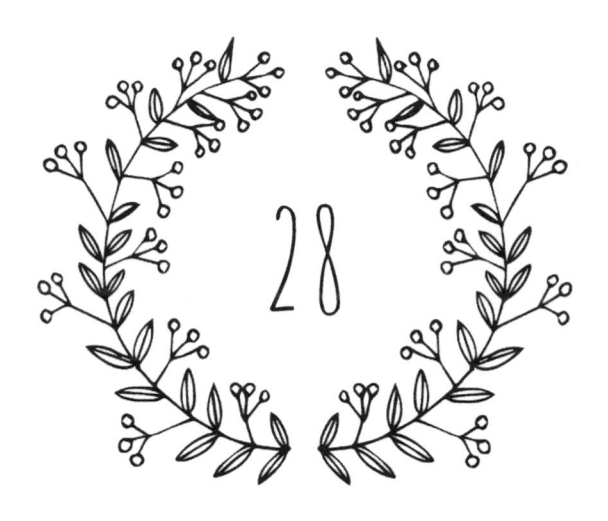

Receive Graciously

What does it mean to receive graciously? It *doesn't* mean drooling and grabbing something out of someone's hands when they give a gift—although it could.

Do you know anyone who doesn't like to receive a gift? I sure don't. Gifts, or money, or favors...it feels great to get happy surprises.

It feels even better if they're things you want or need.

But how does it feel when you get things you don't really want, or like, or care about? Not always great, right? Sometimes you can even feel disappointed.

What do you do in those cases? Do you show your disappointment by handing the gift back and asking the giver to try again? Yikes. I hope not.

Think about how you feel when you give a gift and the receiver is obviously unappreciative, or worse, makes a joke about your gift. Does that really happen?

Yep, it does.

Am I saying you should fake it just to protect the giver's feelings? No. Being inauthentic is never okay. So what do you do if someone gives you a gift you really don't like? What does it mean to receive graciously?

It means to be grateful. Letting people know you appreciate their offerings is actually a way to give back to the giver.

I'm going to tell you something that will allow you to ALWAYS be a truly authentic gracious receiver.

Before you receive a gift, think about the giver. Think about your relationship and the love you share and the caring between you. Reach deep into your heart and receive the love that comes with the gift.

When you do that, it won't matter what the gift is. You'll receive the love.

WHEN PEOPLE GIVE OF THEMSELVES

Do you notice things people do for you? I mean really notice. I'm not asking if you blow things off. But if you're busy, distracted, or not paying attention, things can go unnoticed.

If you don't always notice kindnesses, the person who gives of himself or herself probably notices your lack of acknowledgment. Even when it's a serviceperson on the job and giving is part of their responsibility, people appreciate being appreciated. In fact, most people thrive on appreciation.

Receiving graciously means acknowledging a giver. It means saying "thank you"! And you know what? Your acknowledgment makes the giver want to give more.

Think of yourself. When someone truly appreciates your gift of time or help, doesn't it make you want to keep giving?

Here are a few examples:

> *When a service person tells you to "Have a nice day," say thank you! You don't have to say, "You too." Thanks and a smile will do.*
> *When servers fill your coffee or water glass, even though it's their job, say thank you! (You get more points for making eye contact when you thank them.)*
> *When you put on your turn signal and a driver slows to let you into the lane, acknowledge the person. Wave a thank you!*

What about Compliments?

So I touched a bit on this earlier in the book, but I have a question.

How do you receive compliments? Do you smile and thank the person paying the compliment? Are you embarrassed when people say nice things about you?

Do you deny the compliment and wave it off? Or do you feel the need to return the compliment immediately by saying, "You too," whether you mean it or not?

If you're uncomfortable with receiving, you may not allow others to share your load by giving to you. You may shun offers from people who want to be of service and supportive and tell them you can handle things on your own. Why would you do that? Where might this come from?

How you receive a compliment says a lot about you. Not only does it hint at how you feel about yourself, it also says something about your willingness to receive the goodness life offers.

If you feel uncomfortable accepting offers of support or gifts, it could stem from feelings of unworthiness. Deservingness issues cheat you and the giver out of so much. One of the most valuable gifts you can give someone who cares about you is to receive with grace in your time of need.

Whether compliments, kind words, or gifts, allow yourself to receive graciously, or alternately say no graciously when that's really how you feel.

When you receive graciously, you strengthen your relationships. You connect. Mutual giving and receiving is a beautiful part of life.

I keep a gratitude journal. It's where I track things for which I am grateful, and it helps me avoid taking things for granted. I write out the things I notice during the day, good things that happen and nice things people do for me or say.

Try this! You'll notice opportunities to be grateful all day long. And when you receive graciously, more good things come your way!

Get it done

_____

_____

_____

_____

_____

_____

_____

_____

_____

_____

_____

_____

_____

_____

_____

_____

_____

29

Remember, You're Beautiful

...Just As You Are

As a mother, my primary focus is on giving my kiddos what they need to grow up happy and healthy. It's more important than anything to me. I remind them daily that they're beautiful inside and out, and that they're intelligent and capable and can do ANYTHING they choose.

It's equally important to remind myself of these same things.

Now, I've experienced a ton of success over the last few years and feel pretty confident in my abilities. I DO believe I can do anything I choose to do and I can have anything I want.

I want the same thing for you. Don't be defined by someone else's idea of beauty. I want you to remember you're magnificent, just as you are. You don't have to change for anyone or anything.

You are unique and special and wonderful. But my telling you that means nothing. YOU have to believe it for yourself.

No matter what you have been through in the past and no matter how chaotic your life is today, remembering the beauty you are will get you through to the other side.

Get it done

_____

_____

_____

_____

_____

_____

_____

_____

_____

_____

_____

_____

_____

_____

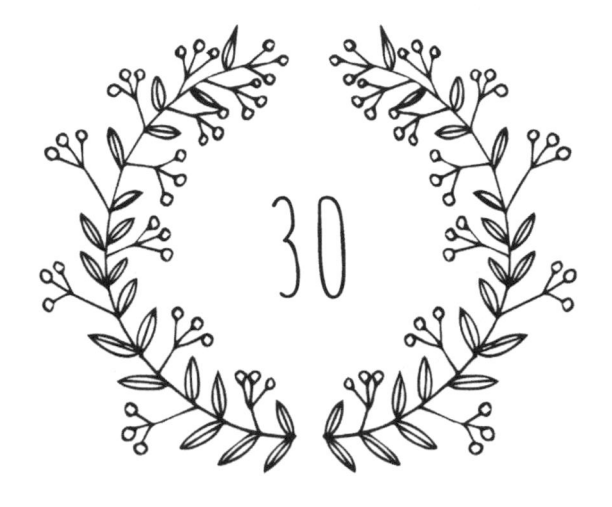

30

Keep Learning

Crack a Book! Take Classes! ...with an Open Mind

You are learning every minute of every day. You absorb so much you are not even aware of most of it. Many people associate learning with traditional education. But if you stop there, that kind of learning pretty much ends after high school or college. By that time, you're just happy it's over so you can move on with your life and start making money.

Okay, so maybe you need a break from formal classroom study. But a commitment to learning in general is mega loaded with benefits that will impact the rest of your life—not just your career.

When I was in law school, I spent hours every day (including weekends) filling my head with knowledge. My course work included exploration of history, politics, and tens of thousands of case studies. Sure, it was a lot of work. I am no longer practicing law, so would I say those years of schooling were wasted? NEVER.

I am so grateful for my education, and I continue to draw on it to this day. You see, once you learn something, you have access to the knowledge forever. It's up to you if you use it and how you use it. You can allow it to fade into your memory bank or you can keep it front and center for the rest of your life. But education and training are never wasted.

Your learning comes from more than academics. It comes from life experience, too. The lessons you learn can catapult you far beyond anything you might ever expect. In fact, one of my friends who is a very successful businesswoman today credits on-the-job learning and life experience for preparing her for success.

Laura always says she learned everything she needed to know about running a successful business working a retail job during college. She learned the importance of good customer service, up-selling, and building relationships—three essential skills for business success. So do not discount your experiences, other jobs, and relationships as sources of success training.

Learning is about more than setting goals, passing tests, and making things happen. It's also about personal growth. None of us knows everything. You'll never know everything, and you can count on things changing once you learn them.

When you commit to learning something new, you're adding knowledge and experience to your skill set. But there's a bonus that comes with tenacity in learning. You have the opportunity to gain a new level of perseverance that benefits future learning. It also keeps your brain young!

There are many levels and types of training. You can take classes at your local community college or adult education program. If you've always been interested in art history, take a course. Learn to cook or take a class that will benefit your business.

Watch webinars. There are tons of free webinars out there! I know, because I devour them on a regular basis. I've also created about a hundred webinars and online courses myself. There's nothing holding you back if you're looking for knowledge or personal development.

Look for podcasts on topics you're interested in. Multitask! Listen while driving or running to double the value of time spent.

Live seminars are another popular vehicle for learning. I like live seminars because I enjoy rubbing shoulders with people and discussing what we're learning. You can learn just as much by listening to other points of view.

There's a flood of information all over the internet, and you can learn volumes simply by Googling a topic! Just be sure not to believe everything you read. Research can be opinionated information, especially when statistics are cited. They can be skewed. You've got a brain—use it.

As an adult, you get to pick and choose the things you want to learn.

Keep filling your head.

Here's why....

- *Learning adds dimension to your life. It makes you well-rounded and keeps your relationships interesting. You'll even make new friends who share your interests.*
- *Learning expands your awareness and helps you adapt to change—something we can count on in today's world.*
- *As learning increases your knowledge, your wisdom expands. The more you know, the more you grow!*
- *Society and technology will continue to evolve and shift. Learning helps you keep pace with those changes and how they affect your own life.*

- *Scientific research says staying active really impacts quality of life. Keeping the brain engaged can help prevent mental and physical ailments. It can delay senior memory issues.*
- *Find something that floats your boat and check it out. Look for classes, seminars, podcasts, and webinars and sign on the dotted line.*

Nope, I'm not done. I have to say one more thing about learning. Time to call forward that inner boss....

Apply what you learn. Don't be the never-ending student who doesn't take action.

There might be fear around things you know you should do, and there will also be things you don't feel like doing. Children often don't want to go to school, but we still send them, right? Guaranteed, when you go to record your first webinar, you will NOT want to do it. But I promise you will not die! And yes, I get it, we all want to do what gives us pleasure and makes us feel good.

Going out there and doing a presentation may not make you feel as good as sitting on the couch eating dark chocolate and potato chips while watching Scandal. Again, you will live. It's just your brain telling you to hide. You need to get out there and DO IT anyway as you'll get nowhere in your life if you only sleep, eat, and hide.

Keep in mind personal experience is the best teacher of all. Your successes and failures have more value than anything you'll watch or read about, but only if you're willing to learn from them. Suck it up, get the lesson, and use it to understand yourself better.

Get it done

_____

_____

_____

_____

_____

_____

_____

_____

_____

_____

_____

_____

_____

_____

_____

_____

31

Follow Your Passion

I'm going to close out our time together with a chapter on following your passion. Why? Because it's what you were born to do. You're here to be you, and if you're not following your passion, you're missing the mark.

Denial of your true self can result in stress. Life does that to get you to pay attention. And if you're not listening, it cranks up the volume.

If you get this one, you'll be less likely to HAVE TO bring yourself back into balance because you'll be there most of the time anyway. Stress will have less impact when you're following your passion.

Your inner boss is strong and courageous. She is uncompromising when she wants something.

Release her. Get clear and follow your passion. If you're following someone else's passion, you will feel it. Don't push that feeling away, because the pain of living for someone else will only intensify until you make a change.

Get in touch with yourself in a big way so you know where to draw the line.

Be honest with yourself. Are you truly happy with your life? Are you doing what you love or doing what someone else wants for you? Maybe you're working for the money. Money is good, but it will not make you happy!

What would you do if your financial needs were taken care of? If you didn't need money, would it be what you're doing now or would it be something different?

There's your answer.

If you would still do what you're doing, you're on the path to following your passion. If you'd quit your job or walk away from your life tomorrow, you're not.

Where are you going from here?

Be realistic. It may not be possible for you to just stop dead in your tracks doing what you're doing. It may take time and planning. But if you're not following your passion, it's time to start taking steps in that direction. You can always take action in one way or another.

Life is too short to live what someone else wants for you—whether it's your family, society, or even your religion. Be clear about what you want and then follow your heart. The answers are there. I promise your heart will never mislead you.

Releasing your inner boss will be easier if you are proactive rather than reactive to what's going on around you. Identify what you want, plan, and then take action. Love yourself enough to understand who you are and why you are here, and then express yourself to the world!

Get it done

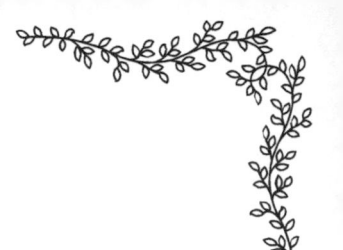

Acknowledgments

Above all, I express my appreciation to my husband, **Wes Hobson**, for his love and support, and to my children, **Makenna** and **Madeline**, for believing in their mamma.

I appreciate...

Amy Porterfield, for waking me up to what was possible, **Kristie Keever**, for her unwavering commitment to me, and **Traci Porterfield,** for helping me make monumental changes in my business.

Judith Cassis, my book coach and editor, for helping me reach deep within to draw out my finest writing, and for never letting me accept second best. I appreciate your unwavering support and creativity.

All my **coaches and mentors;** each of you has helped pave my path to success, and I am deeply grateful for the contributions you've made.

About the Author

Hayley Hobson is an internationally known author and inspirational speaker. Her previous book, *A Beginner's Guide to Essential Oils*, launched in January, 2018.

As a life coach, Hayley passionately empowers others to create lifestyle transformations by supporting clients in becoming the best possible WHOLE versions of themselves. Hayley teaches that consciously creating our thoughts prompts desired results in our personal and business lives. She illustrates her coaching principles in her podcast, *Consciously Creating Your Whole You by Hayley Hobson*, which launched in spring of 2018.

Whether at home in the mountains of Boulder, Colorado, or relaxing at her beach house in Cardiff By The Sea, California, Hayley enjoys spending time with her husband, former world-ranked professional triathlete Wes Hobson, and their two daughters, Makenna and Madeline. Her vegan lifestyle incorporates juicing, fitness, and spirituality.

In addition to Hayley's coaching programs and online courses, she is a sought-after speaker at many global business events. Her programs, presented in more than fifty countries, weave together life coaching principles with strategic business practices.

As a Wellness Advocate, Hayley Hobson is credited with achieving the highest ranks in her company in the shortest time. Today she holds the highest rank of Double Presidential Diamond.

Hayley is an influencer among an expanding network of peers. Her main charitable focus is the building of an orphanage in Haiti that when complete will house up to twenty-five children.

Hayley Hobson has been featured in *The Network Marketing Times*, *The Four-Year Career*, *Positively Positive*, and *Natural Health Magazine*. Her social media following exceeds hundreds of thousands. Look for Hayley on Instagram (@HayleyHobson) and Facebook: https://www.facebook.com/hayleyhobsonwholeyou/

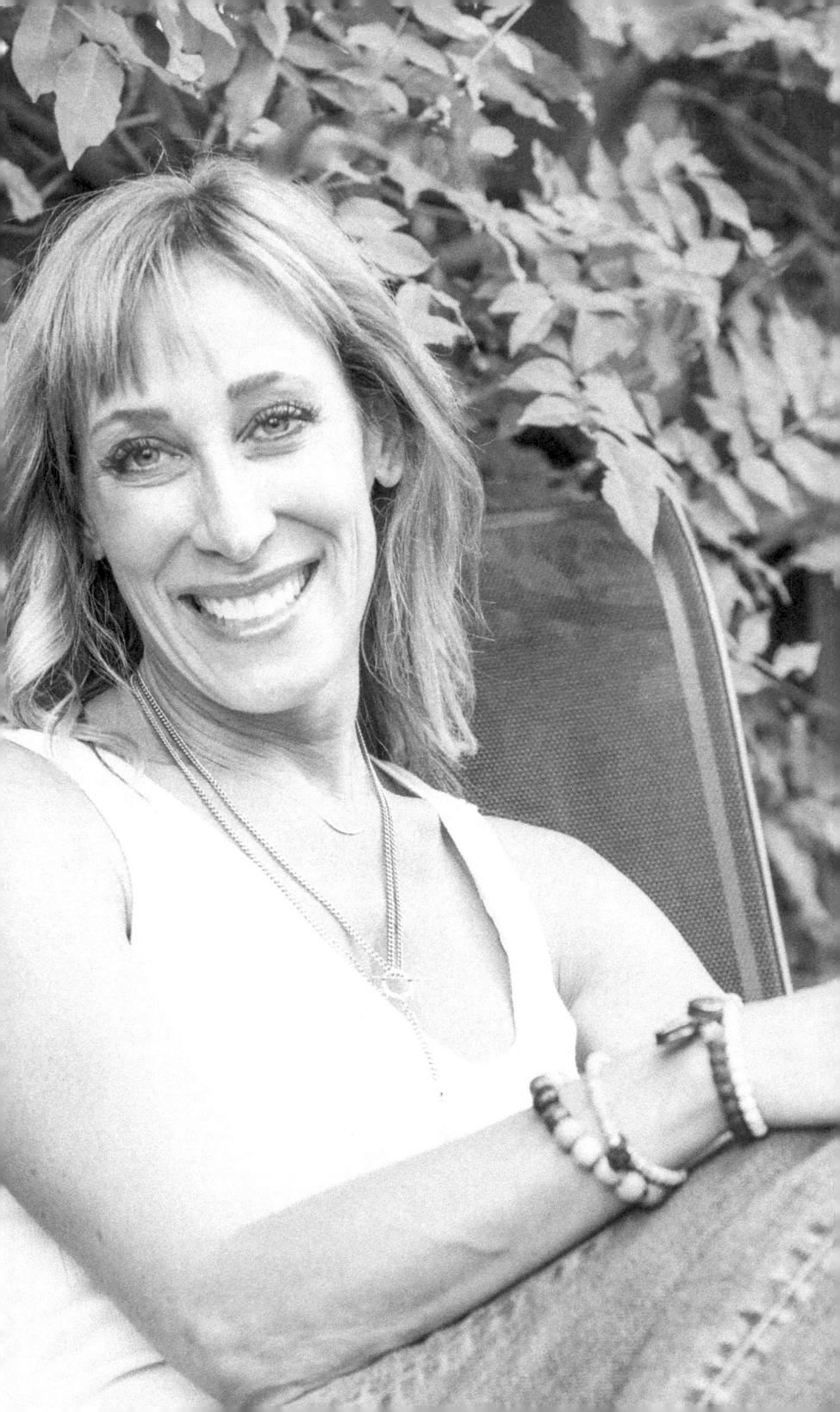

CPSIA information can be obtained
at www.ICGtesting.com
Printed in the USA
BVHW03s1443280718
522902BV00004B/6/P

9 781633 537903